NATURAL
SOLUTIONS
FOR
DIABETES

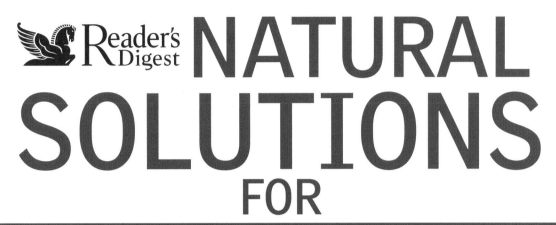

Reader's Digest

NATURAL
SOLUTIONS
FOR
DIABETES

Lose weight & control your condition
ONE STEP AT A TIME

Pat Harper, RD, and Richard Laliberte
with Dr William A Petit Jr, MD

PUBLISHED BY THE READER'S DIGEST ASSOCIATION LIMITED
LONDON • NEW YORK • SYDNEY • MONTREAL

PROJECT STAFF

CONSULTANTS
Azmina Govindji,
Fiona Hunter

PROJECT EDITOR
Caroline Boucher

ART EDITOR
Austin Taylor

RECIPE EDITOR
Norma Macmillan

ASSISTANT EDITOR
Liz Clasen

RESEARCHER
Angelika Romacker

PROOFREADER
Ron Pankhurst

INDEXER
Marie Lorimer

READER'S DIGEST GENERAL BOOKS

EDITORIAL DIRECTOR
Julian Browne

ART DIRECTOR
Nick Clark

MANAGING EDITOR
Alastair Holmes

HEAD OF BOOK DEVELOPMENT
Sarah Bloxham

PICTURE RESOURCE MANAGER
Martin Smith

PRE-PRESS ACCOUNT MANAGER
Penelope Grose

SENIOR PRODUCTION CONTROLLER
Deborah Trott

PRODUCT PRODUCTION MANAGER
Claudette Bramble

READER'S DIGEST USA

EDITOR IN CHIEF AND
PUBLISHING DIRECTOR
Neil Wertheimer

CONSULTANTS
William A Petit Jr, MD
Associate Professor
of Clinical Medicine,
University of Connecticut
School of Medicine; Medical
Director, Joslin Diabetes
Center affiliate at New
Britain General Hospital

Nancy Wright, Certified
Personal Fitness Trainer

Natural Solutions for Diabetes was published by The Reader's Digest Association Limited, 11 Westferry Circus, Canary Wharf, London E14 4HE

We are committed to both the quality of our products and the service we provide to our customers. We value your comments, so please feel free to contact us on **08705 113366** or via our website at: **www.readersdigest.co.uk** If you have any comments or suggestions about the content of our books, email us at: **gbeditorial@readersdigest.co.uk**

Credits
FOOD PHOTOGRAPHY: Sang An, David Bishop, Beatriz daCosta and Elizabeth Watt
EXERCISE PHOTOGRAPHY: Cara Howe/StudioW26
FIRST PERSON PROFILES: Jason Cohn

Book code: 400-272-01
ISBN: 0 276 44087 0
Oracle code: 250009082S.00.24

Acknowledgments

I would first like to thank the Diabetes Obesity Intervention Trial team at the University of Pittsburgh: David Kelley, MD, principal investigator, for his vision, guidance and support; Cindy Kern, RN, project coordinator, for her organizational skills, professionalism and impeccable attention to detail; and Juliet Mancino, MS, RD, for her extraordinary counselling skills and expertise as a diabetes educator. I am also grateful to Judy Arch, RD, and Anne Mathews, MS, RD, for their assistance with this study and their contributions to other weight-loss studies in the division of endocrinology.

I would also like to thank some others who helped me with this book: Nancy Wright, exercise expert and owner of The Wright Fit, for her creativity and expertise in structuring the physical activity recommendations, and Charlene Rainey, of Food-Nutrition Research, Inc., for her invaluable insights. A special thank you to my co-author, Rich Laliberte, whose persistence, patience and talent for writing made the book a reality.

I would especially like to thank the people who volunteered for the DO IT study. Their determination to lose weight by changing their diets, increasing activity and adopting healthier lifestyles was an inspiration to me.

PAT HARPER, RD

Creating this book was a team effort, and my hat is off to my terrific partners, co-author Pat Harper and editor Marianne Wait. Pat is the kind of person you want in your corner when facing a disease like Type 2 diabetes. Her warmth, experience and research skills enable her to get dramatic results without ever forgetting the appeal of a chocolate chip cookie. I'll miss talking to her about the recipes in these pages, when I could almost hear her salivate as she'd say, 'It's really good'.

Marianne kept us on track with her incisive thinking and persistent drive to keep our advice consistent, clear and fresh. Her dedication and high standards made this project the best it could be, and her guidance, comments and laughter are the unsung, invisible heart of the book. I'd also like to thank our medical advisor, William Petit, MD, for clarifying critical questions and ensuring that our plan is safe.

My biggest thanks go to my wife, Rachelle, and our children, Jordan and Marissa, who tolerated several months of deadlines with good humour and were even inspired, like me, to think more critically about what goes on in the family kitchen.

RICHARD LALIBERTE

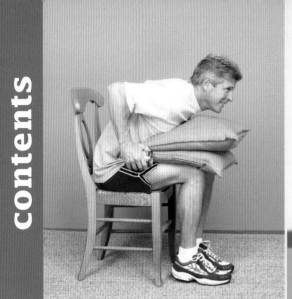
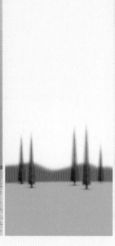
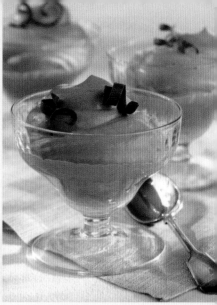

contents

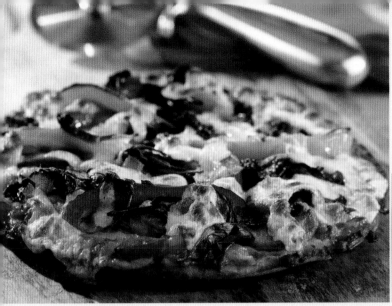
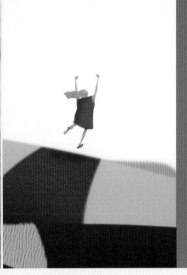

Introduction

SMALL STEPS, BIG RESULTS

Having diabetes need not stop you from living a full life. By managing your blood sugar levels you can still pursue your favourite activities and enjoy delicious foods. That's because, unlike many other chronic diseases, diabetes – particularly Type 2 diabetes – is a condition that's strongly influenced by diet and lifestyle and these are factors that you can control yourself. In fact, research has shown that you can bring down your blood sugar levels significantly simply by adjusting what you eat and how much you exercise.

Perhaps you have tried to change your lifestyle before but not succeeded. You may have started out with the best intentions but soon lost interest. The key to success lies in a simple, practical and achievable plan which this book explains. Its basic premise is straightforward: making one small change at a time is the best way to bring about big results. You may have heard the old saying 'the journey of a thousand miles starts with a single step'. By taking the first step you'll be well on the way to changing your life.

The recommendations made in Natural Solutions for Diabetes are based on extensive research into the effect of diet and lifestyle on blood glucose levels, in particular a study conducted at the University of Pittsburgh School of Medicine in the USA. Here, patients lowered their fasting blood glucose levels significantly just by following a simple plan to help them to lose weight. This wasn't a structured diet; there was no strict calorie counting, nor were there fat targets or banned foods. The idea was not 'to go on a diet' but rather to adopt a healthier lifestyle. This research has formed the basis for the plan in this book, which will help you to reduce your weight by as much as 10 per cent, modify your lifestyle and manage your diabetes in six simple, practical and realistic steps.

Keeping to a well-balanced eating plan is generally recognized as the best and safest way for people with diabetes to lose weight. Some foods have a much greater effect on blood glucose levels and insulin response than others so it is beneficial to include more foods with a low Glycaemic Index (GI) in your diet (see page 64). But the plan in this book allows you to enjoy all food groups and doesn't deprive you of your favourite snacks or desserts. This enables you to enjoy food without feeling restricted, so you are more likely to stick to the plan.

Oversized helpings of calorific food are often the reason we put on weight, but the Plate Approach can change that. This is a visual guide to healthy eating which will help you to cut the number of calories you consume by controlling the size of your portions.

Try out the delicious recipes and the easy and enjoyable exercise routines in this book, and you will soon see the results for yourself. There are also stress-reducing techniques and other lifestyle approaches to boost your energy and lower your blood glucose.

It is important to monitor your progress as you follow the plan. Use the logs and charts at the back of this book to assess how you are changing your diet, how much exercise you are fitting in, how your mood affects what you eat, and how much weight you have lost, then you'll soon begin to see how all of these factors influence your blood glucose levels.

By following the six steps in this plan not only will you lose weight, you may also actually help your body to become less resistant to insulin. And by improving your blood glucose control, you will reduce your risk of complications such as heart attacks, nerve pain, kidney disease and serious eye problems including blindness.

If you can change one small habit today, then another tomorrow, you are in a strong position to manage your diabetes and you'll soon feel better than you have ever felt before. So start with Step One of this plan and consider it your first step towards a healthier, happier, more energetic future.

Azmina Govindji RD
CONSULTANT NUTRITIONIST AND FORMER
CHIEF DIETITIAN TO DIABETES UK

nat

ural

(nat•u•ral) *adjective*

1. Being in accordance with or
determined by nature.

2. Not acquired: INNATE.

3. Without drugs. That's what *we* mean
when we use the word. And believe it
or not, it is possible to control your
blood sugar naturally.

PART ONE
Natural solutions

Introducing
THE
10
Per Cent Plan

You've opened this book for one simple reason. You (or a loved one) have diabetes or a family history of diabetes and you want to manage the condition more effectively. Maybe you'd like to reduce your reliance on medication. Perhaps you're hoping to avoid having to resort to drugs in the first place. Maybe you simply want to do everything in your power to keep your blood sugar under control and to keep serious health problems at bay.

No matter what your situation, if you have Type 2 diabetes, *Natural Solutions for Diabetes* will help you to tame it.

Here you'll discover a remarkably effective approach we call the 10 Per Cent Plan. Follow this plan and you could lower your blood sugar significantly.

You'll also boost your cells' ability to respond to insulin. And you'll do it all with a completely safe, proven plan that will benefit your body from head to toe. Are you ready to take charge of your health?

A new approach to blood sugar control

If you have Type 2 diabetes, your primary goal is simple: to bring your blood sugar levels under control. By doing so, you'll help to stave off diabetes-related complications that can compromise your quality of life, such as serious eye and kidney problems; you can reduce your risk of heart disease (did you know that people with diabetes have two to four times the normal risk of heart disease and stroke?); and you'll most likely live longer. Best of all, you will soon feel better both physically and mentally and more in control of your day-to-day health.

How to lower blood sugar levels is another matter entirely, and one that can seem anything but simple. Medications can achieve this, of course, and you may need to be on some. But there are many more measures that you can take to control your diabetes and slow its progression, starting with changing your diet. There are countless different ways to regulate your diet, from simple healthy eating to choosing the foods you eat according to their Glycaemic Index ratings. But we don't think you should have to research each and every food before you eat it.

This book presents a different idea – a simpler approach. We think that taking charge of diabetes doesn't have to be all that complicated. In fact, it shouldn't be, because the more complicated a piece of advice is, the less likely you are to follow it. Approaches that involve a lot of time, attention and planning can be difficult to stick with permanently.

The truth is that all you really need to do to achieve a radical change in your health is to make a few small changes in some of your everyday habits, such as what you eat for lunch or what you do during the commercial breaks on TV. How can such small changes possibly add up to controlling diabetes? Keep reading, and we'll explain.

Bonus benefits

Lowering your blood sugar levels is reason enough to lose weight for someone with diabetes. But shedding surplus pounds may also help to relieve or prevent a multitude of secondary health problems, including:

- High blood pressure
- Heart disease
- Stroke
- Gallbladder disease
- Joint pain
- Sleep apnoea
- Arthritis
- Breast cancer
- Colon cancer
- Prostate cancer
- Kidney cancer

A WEIGHTY PROBLEM

Most people with Type 2 diabetes have one thing in common: they weigh too much. Britain has the fastest growing rate of obesity in the developed world and, according to a report published by Diabetes UK in March 2005, obese people are up to 80 times more likely to develop Type 2 diabetes than those with a healthy weight. In fact, research shows that being overweight is the single most significant contributor to the development of Type 2 diabetes; so losing weight is the most vital step in bringing it under control (or preventing it).

What does weight have to do with diabetes? Think of excess body fat as a contaminant in your fuel system. Glucose, or blood sugar, is the fuel that powers your body. Normally, glucose, which is derived from the food you eat, has no problem making its way into the body's cells from the bloodstream. But body fat impedes this vital process by releasing substances called free fatty acids into the blood.

Free fatty acids have at least two undesirable effects. One is to cause cells to ignore the glucose and leave it floating in your blood. The other is to cause your pancreas to produce less insulin, a hormone that cells need in order to absorb glucose. So free fatty acids play a major role in diabetes. The havoc that they wreak on glucose absorption and insulin production also contributes to high cholesterol levels, high blood pressure, elevated triglycerides (another type of blood fat) and other problems that may lead to heart disease.

Losing weight is like cleansing your fuel system so that you can use energy more efficiently. The less body fat you have, the fewer fatty acids you will have circulating in your bloodstream, and the lower your blood sugar will be.

The 10 Per Cent Plan

So how much weight do you need to lose in order to lower your blood sugar levels significantly? Perhaps about 20kg (3st 2lb)? Maybe at least 15kg (2st 4lb)? The answer is 10 per cent of what you weigh now – probably much less than you thought. Consider how little 10 per cent is. Ten per cent of an hour is just 6 minutes. Ten per cent of a pizza is barely a slice. And if you currently weigh about 90kg (14st 2lb), 10 per cent is just 9kg (1st 4lb).

Diabetes dictionary

Type 2 diabetes The most common form of diabetes, accounting for about 85 per cent of all cases. The basic problem is that the body's cells are unable to absorb enough glucose, so glucose stays in the blood. In addition, the pancreas may not produce enough insulin, and the insulin may not work properly. This can cause serious complications throughout the body, including heart disease, high blood pressure and kidney, eye and nerve damage. Formerly known as adult-onset diabetes, Type 2 is becoming increasingly common in children, probably linked to rising levels of obesity in young people.

Glucose The body's main source of energy. Glucose, also known as blood sugar, originates in plants and is passed up the food chain. When it accumulates in the bloodstream it makes blood stickier. This makes it more difficult for the blood to flow, which in turn deprives the body of oxygen and nutrients, hinders white blood cells in fighting infection and increases the risk of dangerous blood clot formation.

Insulin A hormone produced in the pancreas that acts like a key, 'unlocking' cells so that glucose can enter. In Type 2 diabetes, the pancreas is unable to keep up with the body's demand for insulin.

Insulin resistance A condition in which the body's cells become less responsive to insulin. Boosting cells' sensitivity to insulin overcomes this resistance.

Fasting blood glucose The amount of glucose in your blood after not eating for 10 to 12 hours. A normal reading is 6.1mmol/l or lower; diabetes is diagnosed at 7mmol/l or higher.

Haemoglobin Alc (HbAlc) A test that indicates what your average blood sugar levels have been over the past two or three months. It measures how much glucose has become attached to the protein haemoglobin, an oxygen-carrying component of red blood cells. The results are expressed as a percentage from 4 to 13. Diabetes UK recommends keeping HbAlc levels below 7.

Hypoglycaemia A condition which occurs when blood sugar levels fall too low, usually as a result of taking too much insulin or going too long without eating. Symptoms include mental confusion, rapid heartbeat, sweating and blurred vision.

A 10 per cent weight loss and the corresponding drop in blood sugar will make you feel better almost immediately – by getting rid of the jittery feelings that blood sugar swings can often cause and giving you more energy, for example. Over the longer term, it will also substantially reduce your risk of diabetes-related health problems, such as poor circulation and kidney damage. Equally important is the fact that losing

10 per cent of your body weight will typically reduce your cholesterol levels, blood pressure and your overall risk of heart disease.

Why 10 per cent? First, because it is relatively easy to achieve. Most university and hospital-based weight-loss programmes produce a 10 per cent weight loss in six months. This is also recommended by Diabetes UK as a 'worthwhile and realistic' target. More important, though, a 10 per cent weight loss is an amount that is virtually guaranteed to lower your blood sugar.

We know that losing 10 per cent has a huge impact because it has been shown to work in studies – not only in overweight people but also specifically in people with Type 2 diabetes. One recent US study took place at the University of Pittsburgh School of Medicine. The goal of the participants was to achieve and maintain a weight loss of at least 7 per cent. What made this study different from others was its approach, particularly regarding eating. *There was no structured diet* – and no carbohydrate counting, food exchanges, specific fat or carbohydrate goals, or banned foods. The idea was to adopt a lifestyle rather than start a 'diet'.

After six months, the participants had actually overshot their weight-loss targets, losing an average of 10 per cent of their body weight, and the resulting reduction in blood sugar levels were even more impressive. The study results were so good that we based our 10 Per Cent Plan on it.

REMARKABLE RESULTS

Participants in the study, officially called the Diabetes Obesity Intervention Trial (DO IT), were given basic dietary guidelines to follow, and then they made their own choices about what to eat. Each week, a dietitian offered suggestions on how to make the meals and snacks they were eating slightly healthier. The idea was to improve the participants' current eating habits here and there, a little at a time, instead of trying to get them to adopt a whole new way of eating. In this book, we'll help you to undertake just such a plan yourself.

The other key component of the study was physical activity. Here, too, the goal was not to start an exercise 'programme' as such, but to introduce more activity into people's everyday routines, starting with small amounts of walking and gradually building more steps into each day.

For six months, the participants went about their normal lives while applying the principles of the plan. Then they went to the clinic for an extensive series of tests and evaluations that required an overnight stay – something they had done at the start of the study as well. One of those tests (not available at your GP's surgery but used by researchers) is for insulin sensitivity, and indicates how well cells are able to use insulin. Six months later the participants returned to the lab again. The results were nothing short of spectacular. By sticking to simple guidelines, the study participants:

- Exceeded the 7 per cent weight-loss goal, losing an average of 10 per cent of body weight after six months.

- Kept weight off through to the end of the year-long study. Although average weight bounced back slightly, on average, the participants were still more than 8 per cent below their starting weights after a year.

- Reduced their fasting blood glucose from an average of 9.4mmol/l – well into dangerously elevated territory – to 6.9mmol/l, which crosses the border into non-diabetes territory. That's a significant 2.5 point difference.

- Brought their haemoglobin A1c levels (a measure of blood glucose averages over a three-month period) down from an

Can you come off your drugs?

For many people on the 10 Per Cent Plan, one of the biggest payoffs will be coming off medication or insulin, or reducing the dosage. We can't make promises. You need to discuss treatment decisions with your doctor, especially when it comes to any changes in drugs. But here's what you might expect if you succeed in bringing your blood sugar down to the following levels:

- **6.1 to 7.8mmol/l** While still above normal, these levels are low enough that you may be able to stop taking all medication.
- **7.8 to 11.1mmol/l** The chances are good that continuing to follow the plan may allow you to come off medication. For now, however, you may still need drugs and perhaps occasional doses of insulin.
- **Above 11.1mmol/l** You may need medication or 24-hour insulin coverage, possibly both, but the plan may enable you to reduce your dosages or make other adjustments. Furthermore, it will most likely lower your blood pressure and improve your cholesterol levels. And of course, you'll enjoy a greater sense of control over your health.

average of 8 (typical for people with diabetes) to 6.7, which is below the goal of 7 recommended by Diabetes UK.

- Improved their insulin sensitivity by fivefold in some cases and, in many cases, by twofold. Because the sophisticated laboratory tests for insulin sensitivity are not generally available you won't be able to check your own sensitivity improvement, but if you have better sugar control with less medication, your sensitivity will have improved.

- Were able to stop taking medication. This was true for 18 of 25 people who were taking drugs at the start of the study.

- Matched the weight loss of a control group that followed the plan and also took the weight-loss drug orlistat (Xenical). By using entirely natural methods, participants in this study achieved the same results as people who tried to get a boost from a weight-loss drug.

Not everyone can expect these exact results, of course. For research purposes, none of the participants weighed more than 136kg (21st 4lb) – the laboratory measuring equipment couldn't cope with people heavier than this. To enable researchers to tell which results came from lifestyle changes, none of the participants was on insulin. Those who were on medication needed to be able to come off their regimens for the study and safely maintain fasting blood glucose levels under 11.1mmol/l – well above the level of 7mmol/l that indicates diabetes, but low enough not to pose acute danger. Regardless of these factors, though, anyone with Type 2 diabetes can significantly benefit from the approach used in the study.

As if the results of the DO IT study aren't impressive enough, there's even *more* you can do to bring blood sugar down naturally and reduce your risk of diabetes-related health problems – and you'll do it on the 10 Per Cent Plan. These measures won't necessarily help you to lose weight, but they will help to lower your blood sugar levels. They include:

- Relaxation techniques which help to improve your glucose control by reducing levels of 'stress hormones' that raise blood sugar.

- Improving sleep patterns and battling sleep deprivation, which has been linked to increased insulin resistance.

Taking the plan on the road

Vince Petroy was ready for a change. At 1m 80cm (5ft 11in), the 58-year-old sales manager tipped the scales at 108kg (17 stone) and had blood sugar levels ranging from 13 to 15.5mmol/l. 'My goal was to stay off medication,' he says. 'I saw my parents taking loads of pills, and I just didn't want to be like that.'

What struck him about the approach of the DO IT study – which is also the approach of the 10 Per Cent Plan – was how easy it is. 'It's very simple, and I followed the guidelines exactly,' he says. 'All it really takes is deciding that you want to be healthy.'

Even though he spends most of his time travelling with members of his sales team, he managed to stick to the plan. In some ways, it even made life easier. 'I'd get jittery when I had blood-sugar swings,' he says. 'And if I was running for a train, I'd just grab a chocolate bar, which made things worse. I found that the best way to control my blood-sugar swings was to make sure I took time throughout the day to eat better foods.' For breakfast, he favoured cereals such as muesli or porridge. Lunch might be a chicken sandwich with a bowl of clear soup. He kept his evening meal light and early. And for snacks he'd have an apple, an orange or a handful of raisins or nuts.

The biggest challenge was taking exercise. 'Initially, it wasn't easy to make myself get out to do the walking,' Petroy says. 'But once I got into the rhythm, I'd feel out of sync if I didn't do it.' While he was on the road, he'd go for a walk as soon as he checked into his hotel. In the morning, he'd get up early and hop on a treadmill in the hotel gym. 'By the end, I was walking an hour a day almost every day of the week,' he says.

His results astonished him. It was as if he were on some miracle drug – but without the drug. After a year, he maintained a weight loss of about 13kg (2 stone) – well over 10 per cent of his starting weight – and had dropped his average blood glucose readings to around 5.5mmol/l. 'My blood sugar levels were absolutely normal,' Petroy says. But that was only the beginning. He also found that he was brimming with energy and slept soundly, without tossing and turning. 'The guys I travel with used to joke, "Has Vince had his nap yet?" They were amazed at my energy once the weight came off. I just feel great. It's been a total win for me.'

● Simple strength-training exercises that build muscle and boost your metabolism so you'll burn more calories.

By incorporating all the elements of the DO IT study plus these extra components, the 10 Per Cent Plan can deliver even more impressive results, increasing your chances of lowering your blood sugar by a significant amount.

WHY THE PLAN WORKS

Many weight-loss plans and programmes for diabetes offer good ideas about what *should* work. What makes the 10 Per Cent Plan so effective? Surveys of participants in the DO IT study and others point to a number of factors that contribute to the plan's power to succeed.

● It corrects simple but fundamental errors committed by many people trying to lose weight, such as going for too long without eating or saving the biggest meal for the end of the day. It also ensures that you cover all your basic nutritional needs without ever feeling hungry.

● It never restricts what you can eat, although you may need to eat favourite foods in smaller portions or prepare them in different ways. A typical comment by DO IT participants is: 'It didn't feel like a diet.'

● It's a plan you can live with. Although recent research has tentatively bolstered weight-loss claims made for popular low-carbohydrate diets – at least in the short term – doctors and dietitians find that many people have an extremely difficult time staying on these diets long term because they are too restrictive. The 10 Per Cent Plan can produce significant results that become a way of life, not merely a temporary fix.

Another important reason to follow this plan is that it has been proven to work for people with Type 2 diabetes. The eating schedule in the 10 Per Cent Plan is specifically designed to keep blood sugar levels from swinging wildly between highs and lows, as well as to reduce your calorie intake so that you lose weight. Unlike many low-carbohydrate diets, the plan steers you clear of the less healthy type of fat that makes blood sugar more difficult to control and raises your risk of heart disease – already a big danger if you have diabetes – and focuses on the 'healthy' fats that facilitate better blood sugar control. You'll be eating unlimited amounts of vegetables, which will provide plenty of the nutrients that people with diabetes need most (not to mention plenty of food, so you won't be hungry). And the exercise you'll take on the plan will help to increase your insulin sensitivity and further decrease your blood sugar levels.

Because the plan doesn't involve maths, it's easy to follow. There's no calorie or carbohydrate counting (except for an initial one-off assessment of your current diet); you don't have to know the specific Glycaemic Index values of all the foods you eat (see page 64); and we won't ask you to eat your burger without a bun or give up potatoes. You're allowed to eat bread and pasta, and even dessert, in reasonable amounts. You will need to make *some* changes – for instance, eat a little less fat, fill your plate with more vegetables, and cut back a little on portion sizes overall – but they aren't big ones. And we know you're ready for change, or you wouldn't be reading this book.

The power of choice

Can a 'self-selected' diet really control blood sugar as well as one that imposes more rigid guidelines? Researchers at Emory University in Atlanta, USA, recently put this question to the test with 648 African-Americans, whose risk of diabetes is twice that of Caucasians. One group of Type 2 diabetes patients was put on an eating plan using food exchanges, while another group was given a much simpler programme that emphasized making healthy choices (balanced meals, less fat) like those of the 10 Per Cent Plan. The result: the people in the healthy choices group improved their blood sugar just as much as those on the plan that used the food exchanges.

Key principles
OF THE
plan

The 10 Per Cent Plan is designed to give you plenty of freedom to decide how you'll meet your weight-loss goal. But that doesn't mean that the plan is completely unstructured or without guidelines. It is actually based on principles that make intuitive sense and are proven to help people with diabetes.

On the 10 Per Cent Plan, we ask you to abide by the following simple rules. Later chapters will give more details on exactly how to do it.

The good news is that you won't be given a list of banned foods, because on this plan all foods are allowed, in appropriate portion sizes. So relax (in fact, relaxation is one of the plan's rules). These are guidelines that will inspire virtually anyone to say, 'Yes, I can do that.'

1 Eat more often

RULE **Start your day by eating breakfast, then go no more than five waking hours without a meal or snack.**

By keeping food in your system, you avoid wild fluctuations in blood sugar – deep valleys brought on by skipping meals or eating them late and high peaks caused by a surge in glucose when you finally get something in your stomach. Just as important, you keep your appetite under control by not letting hunger build to the point where you're ravenous.

Eating more often means, for a start, eating breakfast every day. According to several studies, this not only helps to keep your blood sugar levels stable, it also helps you to eat fewer calories throughout the day. What's more, it boosts your metabolism so you burn more calories.

Research suggests that adopting this simple habit can bring striking health benefits. For example, a report presented to the American Heart Association in 2003 found that rates of obesity and metabolic problems such as insulin resistance were 35 to 50 per cent lower in those who ate breakfast.

In terms of what you eat the rest of the day, if you're planning a late lunch or dinner, you'll need to have a snack in between. That's right, on the 10 Per Cent Plan, we *want* you to snack. Again, the aim is to keep your blood sugar levels steady and make sure you never become too hungry. You'll learn how to master your meal timing in Step One of the plan.

2 Eat balanced meals

RULE **Forget the protein versus carbohydrates debate. We want you to include some of both at each meal, plus at least one fruit or vegetable.**

This is the best approach to controlling your blood sugar, feeling full longer and losing weight. It sounds simple, and it is. Yet clinical experience suggests that if you're overweight, that is probably not the way you're eating now. In fact, your nutritional intake may be so out of balance that you may be deficient in certain nutrients even though you're taking in too many calories. Some nutritionists believe that the body's need for a variety of nutrients triggers your appetite in order to make sure that you get them. But if you simply eat more of what you always eat, your body never gets enough of certain nutrients it really needs. In Step Two of the plan, we show you how to make sure that every meal, whether sit-down or on-the-go, contains the right balance of carbohydrates, protein and fruit and vegetables to keep your blood sugar levels steady and help you to shed pounds.

3 RULE Eat a little less of everything but vegetables

Portion control is essential to weight loss, but that doesn't mean you won't get enough to eat. On the contrary, you have permission to eat as much as you want – of vegetables.

Consider vegetables the ideal food. They are a source of complex carbohydrates and smaller amounts of protein; they are generally low in fat and high in fibre; and they are rich in a variety of vitamins, minerals and other nutrients. That's

Secrets of enjoyable eating

The Food Standards Agency's Balance of Good Health dietary guidelines recommend that you eat a variety of different foods and that you enjoy your food. Provided that you consume a diversity of nutrients and eat food in appropriate portion sizes, spread throughout the day, you can occasionally indulge in your favourite foods. Many nutritionists say it's better to selectively indulge your tastes for richer foods than to condemn yourself to limited choices on a bland, boring diet you'll soon tire of. Here are some ways to increase your pleasure in eating without overindulging.

Slow the pace The best sensual experiences are savoured. By eating more slowly, you deepen your experience of flavours and give your body's appetite controls more time to signal that you're full, so that you ultimately eat less.

Engage the senses You can boost your enjoyment of a meal by appealing to senses other than taste. For example, buy a small bunch of flowers or pick some from your garden to brighten your table; dine by candlelight; or play some of your favourite music at dinnertime.

Indulge yourself Choose one sinfully delicious chocolate instead of a box of fat-free biscuits. The intensity and richness of the treat will make you feel satisfied, and it will actually contain fewer calories than a larger portion of a 'healthier' snack. Just make sure that you have it after a meal rather than on its own.

why different types of vegetables should fill at least half of your plate at any meal. Many fruits offer the same nutritional benefits as vegetables but to avoid getting too many sugars you should limit yourself to three or four portions a day, spaced evenly throughout the day (see page 72).

By adding more vegetables to your plate, you may actually eat more in terms of volume while still helping yourself to lose weight. Plus, you'll leave less room for foods that constitute so much of the typical UK diet: highly processed and packaged foods, meats, sweets, starches and fats. Are these foods forbidden? No. All foods belong in your diet, and everything is allowed. But for the plan to work, your total intake of calories needs to decrease.

In Step Two of the plan, you'll learn how to include more vegetables on your plate. Then Step Three provides menus for breakfast, lunch and dinner, in the correct portion sizes.

RULE 4 ## Trim the fat

Cut back on your total fat intake and substitute healthy fats for not-so-healthy ones.

Fat contains more than double the calories of carbohydrates or protein, so it's an obvious target if you are trying to lose weight. Simply by eating more vegetables, which you will do on the 10 Per Cent Plan, you're likely to eat less fat. But we won't ask you to eliminate all the fat from your diet. In fact, studies show that eating a moderate amount of fat helps people to stick to healthy diets, and some types of fat even help to keep your blood sugar levels steady.

The key is to reduce your intake of the less healthy types of fat by consuming leaner meats and low-fat versions of dairy products, such as milk and cheese. That is because meat and dairy foods contain saturated fats, which contribute to insulin resistance (not to mention clogged arteries). 'Healthy' fats, on the other hand, such as those found in olive oil and in fish, actually help to stabilize your blood sugar because they take longer to digest than carbohydrates.

In one study, women trying to reduce their overall fat intake discovered that their single most effective strategy was to avoid fat as a flavouring – for example, by not slathering butter on bread or potatoes. Instead, use reduced-fat versions of mayonnaise, crème fraîche or salad dressing, or instead of butter use fresh herbs or lemon juice to add flavour. It is also important to include some of your favourite high-fat foods in your diet. In Step Four, you'll trim the fat – and calorie content – of everything from burgers to macaroni cheese. Don't worry, though; they'll still taste great.

5 Take more exercise

RULE **Start to become more physically active by walking – just 10 minutes a day at first. Then gradually build up the time and introduce simple strengthening exercises into your routine.**

Weight-loss experts agree that no weight-loss plan is likely to work unless it includes physical activity. In fact, many of the people in the DO IT study said that boosting their activity levels was one of the most important keys to their success. Exercise burns calories and tones the muscles. It also boosts your muscle cells' insulin sensitivity, making your body more efficient at using glucose and thereby lowering your blood sugar. Furthermore, people who exercise have more success keeping weight off in the long term than people who simply watch what they eat. And exercise feels good. In Step Five, you'll get your body in motion with simple activities such as walking, stretching and gentle strength training.

6 Learn to relax

RULE **Stress not only causes your brow to wrinkle: it also raises your blood sugar levels. We want you to reduce your stress levels using simple relaxation strategies and mood-calming mental techniques.**

When you're feeling stressed, your body releases certain hormones that rev it up and prepare it to fight or flee. The same hormones also raise blood sugar. Recent groundbreaking research shows that you can significantly lower your blood sugar levels by bringing stress under control. In fact, stress-reduction techniques can work almost as well as some diabetes medications. In Step Six, you will learn to manage stress, anxiety and hostility by meditating, breathing, relaxing your muscles and practising mental imagery exercises. We'll also show you how to prevent your emotions from ruling your appetite as well as how to improve your mood – and your blood sugar levels – by getting better quality sleep.

Track your progress

RULE 7

It makes no sense to follow the 10 Per Cent Plan without checking whether it's working. Monitoring your progress will provide encouragement when you see positive results and will highlight any areas where you're struggling so you can work on these.

It's also important to record your efforts to exercise more and eat more healthily. Studies show that people who write down what they eat are more likely to consume fewer calories. And we are convinced that people who track their exercise efforts are more likely to stick to a get-moving plan such as the one in this book.

On pages 208-213, you'll find logs to help you to keep track of your weight, your blood sugar, your exercise and your diet. (You'll read more about tracking your weight and your food intake in the following chapter, 'Before you begin'.)

How often you need to test your blood sugar depends on several factors. You should work out a testing schedule with your doctor. As a general guideline, though, if you don't take medication or insulin and your blood sugar levels stay within a range of between 5mmol/l and 7.2mmol/l, you may be able to restrict testing to just a few times per week. But you should test at least three times a week at the start of the programme, preferably in the morning before you eat anything. Your doctor may also want you to test again before your evening meal for an idea of how your blood sugar level changes during the day.

If your blood sugar swings higher into the abnormal range (above 11.1mmol/l), follow your doctor's advice for testing more frequently. If you're on insulin, medication, or both, you may need to test three or four times a day, typically before meals and perhaps also at bedtime.

Before you
begin

You're probably eager to start the 10 Per Cent Plan immediately. That's terrific, because if you have a positive attitude you're already halfway there. Before you begin, though, take a few minutes to make sure that you are really ready to go.

Here you'll take stock of your current health, determine your weight-loss goal, and analyse your current diet to reveal your biggest pitfalls and discover your best opportunities for improvement.

You'll also find out how to go about following the 10 Per Cent Plan. The answer is by making small changes over time. It's the most effective way to lose weight – and lower your blood sugar – safely and permanently. You can't overhaul your lifestyle overnight, and you shouldn't expect to. Remember, the 10 Per Cent Plan is an approach that you'll adopt for the rest of your life.

Take stock of your health

The 10 Per Cent Plan is for anyone who has Type 2 diabetes or is at risk of it, but, of course, everyone is unique. Your weight-loss target – the number of kilos or pounds you want to lose – will differ from the next person's. Likewise, factors such as whether you are on oral medication or insulin and how long you have had diabetes will influence your goals. One person may set a goal of coming off medication, another may hope to avoid starting medication, and a third may have to remain on medication but want to reduce the dosage. Finally, some people may have health issues that require caution when it comes to certain types of exercise.

Before you start Step One of the 10 Per Cent Plan, take a few minutes to define your weight-loss goals and make sure that you have all the information you need about your blood sugar levels as well as your ability to exercise safely.

Do you have diabetes?

In the UK, 1 million people have diabetes without knowing it. Might you be among them? On average, people have Type 2 diabetes for 5 to 10 years before diagnosis. Warning symptoms include extreme thirst, frequent urination and unexplained weight loss. You are more likely to develop Type 2 diabetes if you:

▸ Have a sibling or a parent with diabetes
▸ Are overweight
▸ Are aged over 40
▸ Had diabetes during pregnancy
▸ Are of Asian or African-Caribbean origin

For an online self-scoring test to assess your risk, go to the American Diabetes Association website at www.diabetes.org

FIND YOUR 10 PER CENT TARGET

First, check what you weigh now. Then calculate your 10 per cent goal by multiplying your current weight in kilograms or stone by 0.1 (if you're calculating in stone, convert your weight to pounds first); that will tell you how much weight you'll aim to lose. For example, if you weigh 100kg (15st 10lb), you'd multiply by 0.1 to get 10kg (1st 8lb). You subtract this number from your current weight to find your target weight. Plan to reach your target weight gradually; your time frame is six months. In most cases, that means losing about half a kilo or a pound per week – a very achievable goal.

Why not aim to lose more than 10 per cent of your weight? Studies find that people who are trying to lose weight often have unrealistic expectations that are self-defeating because they lead to disappointment. By setting a 10 per cent weight-loss goal, you'll have a better chance of succeeding. And it's no small success. Doctors know that the first 5 to 10 per cent of body weight lost has proportionately the biggest effect on blood pressure, cholesterol and glucose levels. See the chart below for a sample of weight-loss goals.

KNOW YOUR BLOOD SUGAR LEVELS

Before you start the 10 Per Cent Plan, book an appointment with your doctor. At the appointment, make sure you get a fasting plasma glucose test to establish your current baseline blood sugar levels. Many people on the 10 Per Cent Plan can expect a drop of about 2.5mmol/l in fasting blood glucose. Depending on where your blood sugar levels are now, that could be enough to get you off medication or even bring your blood sugar back into the normal range.

In addition to the fasting plasma glucose test, you should have a haemoglobin Alc test (abbreviated to HbAlc), which indicates what your average blood sugar levels have been over the past two to three months. If you're not already taking this test every three to six months, you should be. Assuming you have had an HbAlc test within the past three months, and your blood sugar levels and treatment have not changed, use that reading as your baseline for the 10 Per Cent Plan. About three months after you start the plan, have another HbAlc test to get an idea of how your blood sugar levels have changed.

While you are on the plan, it's important to keep close tabs on your blood sugar levels by using a home glucose monitor, not only to see how well the plan is working but also to help prevent a potential side effect of success: hypoglycaemia.

What's your goal?

IF YOU WEIGH (KG)	YOUR TARGET WEIGHT IS	FOR A LOSS OF (KG)
70	63	7
80	72	8
90	81	9
100	90	10
110	99	11
120	108	12
130	117	13
IF YOU WEIGH (ST)		FOR A LOSS OF (ST)
11	9st 13lb	1st 1lb
13	11st 10lb	1st 4lb
15	13st 7lb	1st 7lb
17	15st 4lb	1st 10lb
19	17st 1lb	1st 13lb
21	18st 13lb	2st 1lb
23	20st 10lb	2st 4lb

When you start to lose weight and exercise more, your blood sugar levels will probably drop – after all, that's the point of the plan. But you don't want them to drop dangerously low, especially between meals or after exercise. That's why you should stay in regular contact with your doctor, who will reduce your dose of medication or insulin when it's appropriate.

ASK ABOUT EXERCISE

While you're at the doctor's surgery, discuss your exercise plans. Tell your GP that you'll be walking more in the near future, as well as doing some gentle stretches and strengthening exercises, and ask whether anything about your current health is a cause for concern. For example, if you show signs of poor blood flow or nerve damage (neuropathy), you should pay special attention to your feet, since these problems may mean you're less likely to notice minor injuries that can quickly become serious. This shouldn't necessarily stop you walking, but you may need to take precautions, such as buying a better pair of shoes or using moisturizing cream to help to prevent the skin on your feet from cracking.

People with diabetes also need to be aware of their increased risk of heart problems. Again, light activity such as walking is unlikely to cause any trouble and is actually an excellent way to protect your heart. But if moderate activity causes shortness of breath or chest pain, for example, your doctor may want to follow your progress more closely. You may even be asked to take an exercise stress test before you start exercising if you have diabetes and meet any of the following criteria.

- You're over 35.
- You're over 25 and have had Type 2 diabetes for more than 10 years.

Engineering expectations

Setting your sights on a 10 per cent loss has an advantage over most other weight-loss plans – even those with more ambitious goals. In fact, weight loss is one area in which ambition can work against you. The fact is that many people have unrealistic expectations that can easily lead to disappointment. In one study, researchers asked 60 obese women to define their target weight as well as their 'dream' weight, 'happy' weight, 'acceptable' weight and 'disappointed' weight. In the course of a 48-week weight-loss treatment, the women lost an average of 16kg (2st 7lb) and reported a variety of physical and psychological benefits. Yet almost half had not reached even their 'disappointed' weight, and only 9 per cent had reached their 'happy' weight.

Satisfaction requires a match between what you expect and what you achieve. A realistic short-term goal is to lose half a kilo (a pound) a week. If you succeed, congratulate yourself – then keep going!

- You have any other risk factor for heart disease, such as high blood pressure or high cholesterol levels.
- You've already been diagnosed or show signs of poor blood flow in your limbs, such as pain in your calves or buttocks.
- You've already been diagnosed or show signs of nerve damage, such as tingling or numbness.

Analyse your current diet

'Dear Diary, Today I had one sausage sandwich and a large cup of coffee for breakfast.' These aren't exactly secrets that sizzle off the page, but a food diary *can* make interesting reading (for you, anyway) because it can often be so revealing.

Don't take our word for it. Keep one yourself. It's the only way to get an accurate picture of your eating habits – and that's important to do before you start trying to change them.

Most people think they have a pretty good idea of what they eat. But when it comes to remembering exactly what meals and snacks we've eaten, we're all too prone to forgetfulness. As an experiment, see if you can remember everything you ate in the evening a week ago yesterday. 'Well,' you tell yourself, 'it was a night like any other.' You got home, made your evening meal and relaxed with a magazine. But rewind to making the meal. What if your meal preparations began with opening a packet of crisps? What if you constantly nibbled on the meal ingredients as you put them together? What if you ate the leftovers from the pan in order to avoid washing storage containers? A single week of food diary entries would reveal whether you often eat 'extra' food while preparing meals and uncover those calories that you consume more out of habit than hunger.

The better you understand the way you are really eating at the moment, the better you'll be able to identify your biggest downfalls – and your best opportunities for improvement. If you see in stark figures how many calories you consume in crisps every day, for instance, it's an incentive to switch to fruit, yogurt or pretzels instead. If eating leftovers when washing up after a meal is your Achilles' heel, see it as a great excuse to recruit your children for the chore.

Weight loss is all about choices like these that we make every day, and the choices you *can* make become clearer in light of the choices you *do* make.

WHAT TO RECORD

First, make seven photocopies of the food log on page 210, then use them to keep track of everything you eat for seven days. (That way, you'll be sure to include both weekdays and weekends, when eating habits are often quite different.) You can either carry the form with you wherever you go or use a small notepad to record what you eat when you're not at home, then transfer the information to the form later.

Sample daily food diary

TIME	WHAT I ATE	PORTION	NOTES	KCAL
7am	Coffee with 2 sugars	1 cup	Wake up! Didn't sleep enough	35
7:30am	Cornflakes with	1 bowl	The usual	200
	semi-skimmed milk	1 cup		120
	Orange juice	1 cup		110
8:30am	Éclair		Jim brought a box of	280
			goodies to office	
	Coffee with 2 sugars	1 cup	At desk	35
10am	Coffee with 2 sugars	1 cup	Meeting	35
	Chocolate doughnut	1	Remaining goodies from box	235
			brought to meeting	
1pm	Ham and cheese	1	Lunch	360
	roll with lettuce			
	and 2 slices tomato			
	Small bag crisps	28g		160
	One can of diet cola	330ml		0
3:15pm	Chocolate bar	50g	Hit the vending machine	270
7:30pm	Pizza	3 slices	Too tired and late to	570
			make a real meal	
	Large bottle of beer	330ml		150
7:45pm	Pizza	1 slice	Last piece not worth wrapping	190
10pm	Apple pie with	1 slice	Bedtime snack	395
	vanilla ice cream	2 scoops		265
			TOTAL KCAL	3,410

Don't worry whether your eating fits into a particular meal; just make a note of what you actually put in your mouth – and that means *every* item. Did you grab a handful of raisins on your way out the door? Write it down. Did you take a chocolate from the box when your work colleague passed it round? Did you nibble while preparing the evening meal? Record every morsel. Include beverages and add-ons such as salad dressing, gravy and butter.

It's important to remember that your goal during this for-the-record week is to eat normally. Don't eat as if you're starting a diet or trying to 'be good', even though it may be tempting to make your habits look better than they really are. When you record what you eat, also record:

- The time. This will shed light on patterns in your meals and nibbling.
- Estimated portions. See 'A visual guide to portion sizes' on page 85 for help.
- Notes about circumstances, such as 'popcorn at the cinema' or 'coffee with a neighbour', or how you were feeling, such as 'angry because I got into an argument with my spouse'.

Sample food diary: a quick critique

In the sample food diary on page 33, take a look at the total calorie count. It's about double what it should be if you want to lose weight. Why is it so high? Lunch, for example, is a good, low-calorie choice, as is the diet soft drink. But most of this person's meals and snacks could do with a rethink. These are the problem areas:

- There are few vegetables and whole grains. Apart from lettuce and tomato in the sandwich, this person's choices are almost entirely processed foods with lots of fat, refined carbohydrates, or both. Wholemeal bread would have been a better choice than the roll.
- Each teaspoon of sugar in the coffee adds 16kcal, a total of 96 for the day. Switching to a calorie-free sweetener would save more than 35,000kcal a year.
- This person tends to eat whatever is available – whether it's doughnuts, pizza or a chocolate bar. More careful choices could reduce calories significantly.
- Eating a 25-30g packet of crisps rather than a larger pack is a good strategy, but choosing a lower-fat snack would cut calories.
- Pizza is fine now and then, but this person should have stopped at two slices and could have gained some extra vegetables by adding them on top.
- 10pm is late to be eating more food, especially foods that are high in both calories and fat.

Observations like these reveal your relationship with food and can explain why you eat as well as what and when.

At the end of each day, figure out how many calories each item provided. You can do this by checking the nutrition labels on packaged foods. Be sure to check how many servings the package contains and estimate how much of it you ate. For fresh foods, you'll need a calorie counter – a book that lists thousands of foods and the calories they contain. These are available from bookshops and libraries. For an online calorie counter and lists of popular foods and their calorie content you can log on to a site such as www.weightlossresources.co.uk/calories/calorie_counter.htm.

If calorie counting seems tedious and time-consuming, don't bother with it. The very fact of writing down what and when you eat is valuable even without the calorie counts.

REVIEWING YOUR FOOD DIARY

At the end of the week, put on your detective's hat and look through your diary for clues to your eating habits. The discipline of writing down everything you consumed has probably led you to some surprising conclusions. See if you can detect patterns in your diary – your eating isn't random, even if it feels that way sometimes. Consider the following:

TIME Do you tend to eat late at night or go a long time without eating? (Remember, on the 10 Per Cent Plan, we want you to eat breakfast within 2 hours of getting up and never go more than 5 hours without a meal or small snack. You'll read more about timing in Step One.) Do you eat most of your food in the second half of the day? Does the time of day dictate the food you eat – for example, in the late afternoon are you limited to what's available from the vending machine?

FOODS We often eat without really thinking. You may be convinced that you eat plenty of fresh vegetables and only occasional sweets, but your record may show otherwise. Notice what categories most of your foods fall into. Do you eat a lot of processed foods (foods that come in a box or packet), snack foods, fried foods or takeaways? Do you favour carbohydrates (breads, pasta, rice and cereal) or protein (meat, poultry, cheese and soya products), or do you get some of each at every meal? Do vegetables feature in your food diary? Keep this information in mind. It will come in handy when you read about the 'Plate approach' in Step Two.

ESTIMATED PORTION How much pasta or cereal do you eat at one sitting? Do you tend to go overboard only on certain foods? Do you always finish an item once you've started eating? You may never have thought much about portion sizes before you started your food diary, and perhaps you're eating more than you realized. The key to success depends on eating appropriate portions. On the 10 Per Cent Plan, you'll learn to control the size of your servings. You'll read more about portion sizes – and discover a week's worth of properly portioned meals – in Step Three.

NOTES What's going on – and how do you feel – when you reach for food, especially outside mealtimes? Are you with friends? Watching TV? Stressed out? Bored? In many cases, circumstances have more to do with what, when and how much we eat than whether or not we're hungry. Become aware of situations in which you eat more or eat badly.

CALORIES If you have filled in the calorie column in your food diary take a look at your daily calorie counts. What food accounts for the highest score in your daily tally? Calorie values are hard to guess at because a food's volume has little to do with how many calories it contains. Who would guess that a handful of mixed nuts has the same number of calories as a whole watermelon? Look for high-calorie items that you can trim. You may be surprised by how easy it is to shave substantial calories from the choices you typically make. Let's say fried chicken is one of your favourite dishes. Simply by switching from a fried chicken thigh (240kcal) to a roasted skinless chicken breast (140kcal), you'll save 100kcal. On the 10 Per Cent Plan, you'll learn many ways to trim your total calorie intake, sometimes by preparing a food differently and sometimes by eating a little less of it.

We won't ask you to hit a particular calorie goal on the plan, but if you want to know how your current calorie intake compares with recommended targets for weight loss, women who are trying to lose weight are typically advised to limit their intake to around 1,400kcal a day, and men are advised to limit their daily intake to between 1,600 and 1,800kcal.

Quiz
Analysing your food diary

Check your food diary to help you to answer the following questions. For each, circle the number to the left of the answer that best reflects your choices.

1. I eat breakfast:
1 Hardly ever
2 Off and on
3 Every day

2. Between meals, I:
1 Don't eat anything at all
2 Always have at least one large snack
3 Have a light snack if I feel hungry

3. I eat the most:
1 At my evening meal and throughout the evening
2 At lunch and throughout the afternoon
3 In the morning and at lunch

4. At lunch and dinner, I:
1 Rarely eat vegetables with my meal
2 Sometimes have a vegetable
3 Almost always have at least one vegetable or a salad

5. I eat fruit:
1 Seldom
2 A few times a week
3 One to three times a day

6. When I eat a carbohydrate food, it tends to be:
1 Chips or sugared cereals
2 White bread, pasta, white rice or mashed potatoes
3 Whole grain breads and cereals or starchy beans, such as kidney beans or other pulses

7. Most of the foods I eat tend to be:
1 Fast food or takeaway (Chinese, Indian, pizza)
2 Processed foods (packaged foods, ready meals)
3 Fresh (fruit, vegetables, meals cooked at home using fresh ingredients)

8. My biggest sources of calories are:
1 Desserts or snack foods
2 Meat and potatoes
3 Vegetables, fruits and whole grains

9. When I drink beverages, I prefer:
1 Regular soft drinks
2 Fruit juice
3 Diet drinks or water

10. I eat sugary foods such as biscuits, cakes and sweets:
1 More than once a day
2 About once a day
3 Less than once a day

11. The meats I eat the most tend to be:
1 Processed meats such as burgers, sausages or canned meat
2 Chicken with skin on, lamb, fatty cuts of meat or minced beef
3 Skinless chicken, extra-lean mince, lean beef, pork or ham

12. My meals consist of the same foods:
1 Four or more times a week
2 Three times a week
3 Once or twice a week or less

Add up your score, then turn the page.

Quiz
What your score means

27 to 36 Your eating habits are already pretty good. So why are you overweight? The chances are, your portion sizes are too big (see Step Three) or you are not taking enough exercise (see Step Five).

18 to 26 You're off to a good start, but your eating habits could do with some improvement. What changes should you make? Look back at your answers. Did you circle any 1s? Read through the comments on those questions below to see how the 10 Per Cent Plan will help you.

12 to 17 You tend to make poor food choices, but that means you have the most to gain from even small improvements. Review your answers. Did you answer any with 3s or 2s? These are successes: give yourself credit, and make more 3s and 2s your goal.

The logic behind the questions

1. Research shows that people who eat breakfast have greater success at losing weight – and the right breakfast will help to keep your blood sugar levels steady for hours.

2. Going without food for more than five hours makes you ravenous and leads to overeating. You'll learn that it's fine to snack between meals if you keep portions small.

3. Having a big evening meal and eating late at night piles on calories when your metabolism is slowest. It's better to get most of your calories early in the day.

4. Vegetables will fill the biggest part of your plate in the 10 Per Cent Plan because they are highly nutritious and filling and yet don't contain many calories.

5. Fruits provide plenty of nutrients and fibre, so it's good to eat some daily. Because fruits have more calories and sugar than vegetables, you should eat vegetables more often.

6. Carbohydrates are not necessarily bad for people with diabetes, but some carbohydrates are better than others. Whole grains and beans help to steady your blood sugar levels, while refined carbohydrates (white bread, refined breakfast cereals) and sugar cause levels to fluctuate.

7. Fresh foods tend to contain more nutrients and far less fat, calories and sodium than processed or fast food.

8. Knowing the sources of your biggest calorie intakes is your first step towards cutting back on foods that put on pounds.

9. Beverages – even fruit juice – can be a surprisingly significant source of calories. Switching to diet drinks or water can make a big difference to your waistline.

10. Desserts are fine, in small amounts. We'll help you to switch to lower-sugar desserts and healthier snacks.

11. Some meats are very high in fat. Choosing leaner cuts saves you calories and cuts back on saturated fat – the kind that decreases insulin sensitivity.

12. Variety is the spice of life. If you eat the same things over and over again, you should make sure they're good for you. It's preferable to vary your meals as much as possible.

Following the 10 Per Cent Plan

By now, you probably have a pretty good idea of what to expect on the 10 Per Cent Plan. Maybe you're asking yourself, 'When do I start?' and 'When do the payoffs begin?' The answer to both questions is today.

On the 10 Per Cent Plan, each day should be a small victory – and each small victory should bolster your efforts to achieve another. Soon – how soon depends on you – those little triumphs will start to show up on the scales and in your blood sugar readings.

There's no set timetable on the 10 Per Cent Plan and no pressure to shed huge amounts of weight at once. In fact, we don't want you to rush into making big changes. Instead, the idea is to make slow and steady progress at a pace that seems right for you.

Start by making one change – such as eating whole grain cereal for breakfast or having more vegetables at dinner – and try to stick with that new habit for a few days, a week, or even two weeks before you attempt to make another change. Each planned improvement in your eating or exercise habits should make you think, 'That's no big deal.' Can you eat a mini-muffin instead of a full-size one? (No problem.) Can you take a 10-minute stroll most days? (Don't see why not.) Can you throw a handful of frozen mixed vegetables into your soup? (You call this a diet?) Changes like these can – and should – seem almost trivial. But as you keep building on them they add up to differences that are truly significant.

This is a radically different approach from weight-loss plans that make you change your eating habits overnight. We don't need to cite studies (although there are plenty of them) to show what you probably know from your own experience: dramatic diets can produce dramatic results, but they involve too much hard work. You soon tire of them and go back to your old ways – and those dramatic results quickly evaporate.

The 10 Per Cent Plan, on the other hand, provides a solution for life. It starts with what you eat now and how much you currently exercise, then makes small tweaks here and there – and keeps making them – until you have lost weight and lowered your blood sugar. How could one change make you lose weight? The answer is, it won't – by itself. But that one change (eating strawberries with yogurt instead of ice cream, for example) will *start* to make you lose weight. With each passing day, you'll feel more successful and motivated, and you'll be able to compound your efforts with more changes. It's like a bank account that starts with just £1 and doubles every day. In 21 days, that pound makes you a millionaire.

What happens after you have lost 10 per cent of your body weight? Nothing changes. You keep on doing exactly what you have been doing. If you want to lose more weight, you can look for additional small victories to win based on the principles of the 10 Per Cent Plan.

We have organized the plan into steps, but there's no real need to follow them in sequence. If you're willing to start walking tomorrow, feel free to skip ahead to Step Five. If stress-related eating is a major problem for you, you may want to start with Step Six. And if you start at the beginning with Step One, you'll find 'fast track' tips (such as those on the opposite page) to give you a head-start on the steps to come.

TRACKING YOUR WEIGHT

While you're on the 10 Per Cent Plan, you will want to weigh yourself consistently and accurately to monitor your weight loss. The best approach is as follows.

- Weigh yourself in the morning. Weight can fluctuate by as much as 2.5kg (5lb) during the course of a day. Your weight is most accurately determined first thing in the morning, after you've been to the toilet but before you've eaten or dressed.

- Weigh yourself only once a week. Your weight fluctuates from day to day so it is not helpful to weigh yourself more often than this.

- Expect progress to vary. Clinical studies suggest that after four to five weeks of steady losses, your weight might increase by about half a kilo (one pound). Thereafter, the pattern is likely to be one of losses followed by smaller upward blips. Don't be discouraged by these periodic gains as your metabolism adjusts: they are quite normal. Look at the big picture. If the overall weight trend is down, you're succeeding.

On the 10 Per Cent Plan, you'll eat a little less, never allow yourself to become too hungry, and introduce more physical activity into your day. To see how easy it can be, do these four things today.

Eat a high-fibre breakfast

Breakfast is a crucial element of the plan because research suggests that people who start the day with a well-balanced meal do better at controlling blood sugar and losing weight. The best breakfasts contain significant amounts of fibre, which slows digestion, helps you to feel full on fewer calories and slows the rise of blood sugar after a meal. Try one of these:

- 3 tbsp wholegrain cereal mixed with 75g (2½ oz) sliced strawberries, 25g (1oz) chopped ready-to-eat dried apricots and 175ml (6fl oz) semi-skimmed milk (4g fibre, 300kcal).

- 200ml (7fl oz) low-fat yogurt mixed with 2 tbsp sugar-free muesli and a handful of fresh blueberries (3g fibre, 250kcal).

- 2 slices wholemeal toast topped with 2 tbsp wholenut peanut butter and 1 mashed medium-sized banana (5g fibre, 350kcal).

Take a 5-minute walk

You don't need to set aside an hour a day for a workout in order to start becoming more active. All it takes is a commitment of 5 minutes a day – long enough for a short walk. Small jaunts fit easily into daily life and require so little time, they are hardly a big commitment. Yet the mere act of putting one foot in front of the other gets you in the habit of moving. You could, for example:

- Get off the bus one stop early and walk the rest of the way home or to work.

- Go for a short walk in your lunch hour or after your evening meal.

- Use the stairs rather than the lift or the escalator.

Check the TV listings

People in the UK watch on average 2½ hours of television a day, and most of us find ourselves glued to the box simply because it happens to be on. Check the TV listings and decide what you want to see, then watch only that programme. This should free up substantial chunks of time that you can use for more active pursuits. The link between TV viewing and weight is striking. A recent Harvard study of 68,000 women showed that those who regularly watched 2 hours of TV a day increased their risk of becoming obese by 23 per cent and of developing diabetes by 14 per cent.

Select one food and eat a little less of it

For weight loss, what you eat may matter less than how much of it you eat. With the 10 Per Cent Plan, you will aim to consume fewer calories than you do now. You can do this by making substitutions, but you can also reduce your calorie intake by simply eating less of foods. If you love bacon, for example, choose lean back instead of streaky bacon and eat two rashers instead of three.

It's also important to bear in mind that if you have started to exercise more (as you will when you get to Step Five), you may be building up muscle, which weighs more than fat. So although your clothes may start to fit better and your trousers fasten more easily, you may not immediately notice much difference on the scales. Be patient. Muscle burns energy faster than other types of tissue (especially fat) so building up muscle means you'll burn more calories and ultimately lose more weight.

ADJUSTING YOUR MEDICATION

If you're currently on medication to bring down your blood sugar, you'll probably be able to adjust your dosage once you start to lose weight. Of course, you'll need to make that decision in consultation with your doctor. As you proceed with the plan, monitor your blood sugar regularly and inform your doctor of any changes. (If you don't already have a blood sugar log, use the one on page 213.)

Are you ready?

If you're trying to lose weight now you've probably tried to do so before. Studies show that the attitudes and psychological baggage you carry from previous attempts can affect how well you do today – if you allow them to. Do you have the right attitude to succeed? Look at the checklist below and tick all the statements you agree with.

❏ The best way to lose weight is slowly and gradually, not all at once.

❏ Achieving a weight loss of 10 per cent is a major accomplishment that will have a significant impact on my health.

❏ I'm willing to make small adjustments in my dietary habits as long as I can eat foods I like.

❏ I'm certain there are ways I can work more physical activity into my life without too much trouble.

❏ Two steps forward and one step back is still progress.

❏ I don't want to be on a diet – I want to permanently change the way I eat.

❏ Diets haven't worked for me, but it's still possible for me to lose weight.

The more ticks you placed next to these statements, the more certain you can be that you have the right mental attitude to make this plan work for you. The next question is when to start – but that implies that you need to wait for the sound of a starter's pistol or the word 'Go!' for permission to cross the line. Don't wait. You can begin making small changes *straight away*.

Beyond saving money and sparing you potential side effects, cutting back on medication may actually help you to lose weight. This is because losing weight and taking more exercise will cause your blood sugar to drop. If you don't lower your medication dosage, your glucose levels may drop so low that you'll be tempted to overeat.

How you adjust your medication will depend on how much your blood sugar levels vary, your history of hypoglycaemia, the type and dosage of your medications and how much you are exercising. As a rule, moderate exercise is unlikely to cause blood sugar levels to plummet, but it's not uncommon for exercisers at the start of a programme to feel 'shaky' or 'weird' after a bout of activity. These effects can easily be overcome by eating a small amount of a sugary food, such as a square of chocolate, drinking a small glass of fruit juice, or taking a glucose tablet made for this purpose. But there's a natural tendency to take this 'permission' to eat a little too far – by having, say, a whole piece of pie or an entire meal – and that won't do your weight-loss efforts any good.

CONTINUING YOUR FOOD DIARY

We won't insist that you keep a food diary indefinitely, but if you're serious about succeeding, it's something you should consider. Studies have shown that people who continually monitor their eating habits – in writing – are more likely to eat fewer calories and lose weight than those who don't. And in cases where both record keepers and non-record keepers shed pounds, the note takers lose more.

'Even when travelling, I'd carry a piece of paper in my jacket pocket to write on,' says sales manager Vince Petroy, who lowered his blood sugar to normal levels from highs of above 15mmol/l during the DO IT study. 'I'd jot down what I ate and fill in the log later in my hotel room. It wasn't a big deal. In fact, it was a good talking point.'

If you hate the idea of keeping a food log, and it becomes an obstacle to your staying on the 10 Per Cent Plan, it's better to ditch the diary. But even writing down what you eat 50 to 75 per cent of the time has been shown to make a measurable difference in weight loss.

solu

tion

(so•lu•tion) *noun*

1. A homogeneous mixture of
two or more substances.

2. A set of values that satisfies
an equation.

3. The answer to a problem.
The 10 Per Cent Plan is your
solution to high blood sugar.

PART TWO

The 10 Per Cent Plan

STEP 1 Master your timing

It's true in love, war, business, comedy – and weight loss: timing is everything. Simply by watching when you eat, you can go a long way towards stabilizing your blood sugar as well as preventing your body from storing food as fat.

The beauty of the 10 Per Cent Plan is that we want you to eat more often, not less.

Contrary to what you might think, it is the best way to lose weight, and it helps to keep glucose swings in check. So don't be tempted to skip breakfast. And feel free to eat snacks.

When you have diabetes, eating is a little like a ride on a roller coaster. Meals spaced far apart are the scariest coasters, with steep climbs followed by huge drops. By eating more frequently, the peaks are lower and the troughs are shallower – closer to what people with normal blood sugar experience. It's an easy way to feel better, weigh less and take charge of your diabetes.

Most diet plans focus on *what* you eat. With the 10 Per Cent Plan, we want you to think first about *when* you eat. You may not think of timing as a critical part of a successful weight-loss plan – and that's why it is often overlooked. Poor timing of meals is one of the biggest trouble spots for overweight people with diabetes. But luckily it's an easy problem to correct.

Why is timing so crucial? Consider the typical approach to slimming down. If you want to reduce your calorie intake, the reasoning goes, you should eat less often since fewer meals mean less food. But the logic is flawed. Skipping meals or going for long periods without eating will backfire in the long run. That has been proven in studies and large surveys, and you may even have discovered it first hand. It's true that eating less often means that you temporarily avoid calories you would otherwise have eaten – but those calories tend to show up with a vengeance when you become so hungry that you eat everything in sight. In addition, and just as important for people with diabetes, missing meals makes your blood sugar levels fluctuate more erratically. That's why two fundamental rules of this plan are:

Help!

My blood sugar level is sky-high in the morning. Shouldn't I skip breakfast to bring it down?

No. It's true that for some people with diabetes blood sugar tends to be high in the morning. That's because as dawn approaches, your body starts to release energizing hormones to rev you up for the day. These antagonize the action of insulin and stimulate the liver to produce more glucose, even if the glucose level in the blood is already abnormally high. Will eating push it up even higher? Probably, but because breakfast is important for proper nutrition and weight loss, you need to make it a priority and find other ways to deal with the 'dawn phenomenon'.

Start checking your blood sugar at 7am. If it is often above 11.1mmol/l, try controlling the morning spikes by taking action the night before. For instance, you could eat less in the evening or try exercising before you go to bed, which siphons glucose from the blood into the muscles for hours afterwards. If you're taking insulin, your doctor may need to adjust the timing or amount of your last dose of the day. Or you may need a morning dose of medication (taken with food) to help keep your blood sugar under control until proper eating, exercise and stress management get you on a more even keel.

- Eat within two hours of getting up each morning.

- Go no more than five hours without eating a meal or light snack.

If you are a person who rushes out of the door without eating anything in the morning or allows yourself to go so long without eating that your stomach rumbles and growls for food, you need to pay particular attention to this advice.

Treat yourself to breakfast

Begin with the first rule: eat within two hours of getting up. Actually, the two-hour mark is pushing it – that is the absolute maximum amount of time you should wait before eating. It's a better strategy to set a goal to eat within the first hour, and then you will have an extra hour of leeway if your morning gets out of control.

Research findings have linked eating breakfast with lower rates of both obesity and insulin resistance. A recent Nottingham University study of lean, healthy women found that skipping breakfast raised their cholesterol levels and reduced their bodies' sensitivity to insulin. The women also increased their calorie intake on breakfast-free days.

Starting your day with something to eat is a good idea even if you don't have diabetes or need to lose weight. The most obvious reason is that your body needs fuel after going many hours without nourishment, and eating breakfast provides that fuel so that you feel more energetic and alert. But in addition, getting breakfast into your system stokes up your calorie-burning furnace and keeps it burning hot throughout the morning. Otherwise, it will stay on 'low' because your body turns it down while you sleep so as to conserve energy. Eating breakfast gives your body permission to turn up the thermostat so you burn the calories from your morning meal (assuming the portions are reasonable; we'll cover this in more detail in Step Three), and the coals stay hot so you are more likely to burn stored fat.

Eating a healthy breakfast – especially one that contains whole grains, such as wheat or bran cereal, muesli or porridge – also seems to make it easier for people to resist fatty and high-calorie foods and therefore more likely to stick to a healthy-

Shake breakfast up

If you're someone who can't face eating much in the morning and finds it difficult to get over the hurdle of making morning meals a habit, why not whip up a healthy shake or smoothie? Refreshing and nutritious, they also are quick to prepare. All you need is a sharp knife and a blender or food processor. But limit the amount you drink to 300ml per day.

Fruit (fresh, frozen, dried or canned) combined with milk and/or yogurt are the main constituents of most shakes or smoothies, but you can add other ingredients, such as wheatgerm or nuts, to boost their nutritional value.

If you decide to use canned fruit, choose fruit in natural juice or water rather than in syrup. Frozen fruit makes a good alternative to fresh fruit, particularly during the winter months, and it gives smoothies a thick, creamy consistency.

Choose skimmed or semi-skimmed milk and low-fat yogurt in preference to the full-fat versions.

An ultra-fast breakfast

Got a minute? That's about all you need to prepare a hot egg sandwich for a speedy breakfast before you leave home in the morning. Here's how.

▸ Break an egg into a saucer and whisk it with a fork.

▸ Microwave the egg on high for 30 seconds. Take it out and whisk again to keep the edges from overcooking, then microwave it for another 30 seconds.

▸ Serve your perfectly formed egg on toast. Note: you will need to pop the bread into the toaster before starting the egg, so they are ready at the same time.

eating plan. According to the US National Weight Control Registry, a survey of successful dieters, an impressive 78 per cent say they eat breakfast every day, while only a minuscule 4 per cent say they never do.

BREAKING IN A BREAKFAST ROUTINE

If you're not accustomed to eating in the morning, relax. Breakfast is easier to prepare than any other meal. There's no need to dig out the frying pan for a breakfast of eggs and bacon or pancakes. (Those aren't ideal breakfast foods anyway – although you can have them if they are prepared and portioned to keep calories low.) In fact, the simpler you keep breakfast, the more likely you'll be to eat the best kinds of foods, such as raw fruit and whole grain cereals. So how do you start?

PUT EATING FIRST Try to have breakfast shortly after you get out of bed. That way, you'll eat before you remember that you have to take out the rubbish, walk the dog, pay bills or do any other distracting tasks that can gobble up your time.

GIVE YOURSELF TIME You may be skipping breakfast more out of a frantic need to beat the clock than from a misguided desire to avoid calories. A simple way to ensure you have time to eat is to set your alarm 15 minutes earlier. But be sure to go to bed at least 15 minutes earlier at night. The last thing you want to do when you have diabetes is to shortchange yourself on sleep (we'll cover this in more detail in Step Six). If possible, try to get up before the rest of the family. It's easier to make sure you feed yourself when you don't have to deal with children, live-in parents, spouses or others who may demand your time and attention.

TAKE IT WITH YOU If you find that it's simply impossible to fit in a sit-down breakfast before you leave home in the morning, don't despair. There are plenty of foods that are perfect for carrying in your bag or briefcase (see the 'Grab-and-go menu' below).

REDEFINE BREAKFAST Some people with diabetes say that they just don't like breakfast. In the majority of cases, what they really mean is that they don't like traditional breakfast foods. But who says that breakfast has to be eggs, toast or cereal? As long as your body has a mixture of protein and carbohydrate, it doesn't matter what you eat. Here are some examples of breakfasts that are just as nutritious, balanced and low in calories as cereal and milk.

- Wholemeal toast spread with peanut butter and topped with a mashed banana

- Oatcakes spread with reduced-fat soft cheese

- Baked beans on wholemeal toast

- An egg salad sandwich made with a wholegrain English muffin

PREPARE THE EVENING BEFORE Your mornings may well be a hectic rush. But that's no reason to skip breakfast. A good strategy is to start preparing the night before. To save precious minutes in the morning, try adopting any of these evening approaches.

- If you have a coffeemaker with a timer, remember to fill it and set it for the desired time. Otherwise, fill your coffee machine in the evening so that all you have to do in the morning is turn it on and wait for it to brew.

Grab-and-go menu

Even when you're eating on the go, it is possible to have a balanced meal that includes protein, carbohydrate and a fruit or vegetable. (You'll find out much more about the importance of this balance in Step Two.) You can accomplish a balanced meal with these combinations of foods.

PROTEIN	CARBOHYDRATE	FRUIT
1 hard-boiled egg	1 small low-fat wholemeal muffin	1 medium banana
25g (1oz) reduced fat cheese	1 mini-bagel	1 medium apple
200ml (7fl oz) low-fat milk	1 cereal bar	20 seedless grapes
200ml (7fl oz) low-fat yogurt	2-3tbsp breakfast cereal	50g (2oz) raisins
25g (1oz) bag mixed nuts	2 oatcakes	175ml (6fl oz) juice

- Set out plates, bowls, cutlery and nonperishable foods such as cereal and breakfast muffins so they will be ready when you are.

- Hard-boil eggs and put them in the refrigerator.

- Do chores that you normally save until morning, such as putting out the rubbish, making packed lunches, or emptying the dishwasher. (This may have the added advantage of helping to prevent you from snacking at night.)

- Cut up fruit that you can spoon into a bowl with your cereal for an instant breakfast. Cover and refrigerate overnight.

Upstage your appetite

As a rule, people who eat small amounts all day long tend to consume less when they finally sit down to a real meal. But that is not always the case. If you still find yourself eating huge dinners, try eating a small part of the meal – such as a slice of low-fat cheese – about 20 minutes before you sit down. That's how long it takes for your brain to register the food and trigger a feeling of 'fullness'. The pre-meal snack will reduce the urge to overeat at the table.

Eat between meals

'Don't eat between meals.' 'Don't spoil your appetite.' You have probably had these messages drummed into you since you were a child, and may even have passed them on to your own children. But just because they are repeated so often doesn't make them true.

Before you leave home in the morning, think ahead to when you're likely to eat again. The chances are, it won't be until past noon or 1pm. If you have breakfast at 7am, that's more than five hours between meals – and that's too long. The solution is to have a light snack around mid-morning. This means that unless healthy foods are easy to find wherever you are during the day, you will need to pack your snack before you leave the house.

Why do you need a snack? It takes about four hours to digest a meal – five hours at the most. After five hours, your stomach is completely empty, and your intricately tuned metabolism starts to respond accordingly. Is more food on the way? Your body has no way of knowing. You might assume that it starts tapping the body's store of fat for fuel as a result, but what mainly happens is that it begins to slow your metabolism to conserve energy. That makes it harder to burn fat, not easier. It's similar to what happens when the fuel gauge on your car drops into the red zone. When you think you're virtually out of fuel you ease up on the accelerator.

After lunch, the story is the same. If you won't be eating again for five hours or more, be sure to have a snack about halfway between lunch and your evening meal.

Some nutrition researchers estimate that spreading your calories throughout the day instead of heaping them on in big meals makes the body burn as many as 10 per cent more calories. Just as important, it prevents major hunger pangs that make you want to eat everything in sight. No wonder a study conducted at the University of Massachusetts Medical Center in 2003 found that people who ate four times a day were 45 per cent less likely to be obese than people who ate three times or less. Other studies support the notion that eating more often facilitates weight loss.

Curb night-time calories

Now for a final guideline: try to eat your last meal of the day no later than 7pm. In a sense, mastering your food timing throughout the day is all about meeting this last goal, because it helps solve a big problem that is common among people with diabetes: eating – and overeating – at night. That's when most of us have more time to sit down for a big meal. Then we turn on the television and continue to eat. If this describes you, you're not alone. Many overweight people with diabetes eat more calories at night than at any other time of day.

A large intake of calories is exactly the opposite of what you really need, however. At night, your metabolism winds down as your body prepares for sleep. In terms of physiology, this is when your body needs

Right-sizing your snacks

The only problem with snacks is that they can become more like additional meals if you go overboard. If you're careful, though, there's no reason why snacking can't be both light and satisfying. As a guideline, you should limit each snack to no more than 150kcal. Good choices that fit the bill include:

▸ 200ml (7fl oz) low-fat yogurt

▸ 25g (1oz) cheese

▸ 1 oatcake or rye cracker spread with reduced-fat soft cheese

▸ A handful of cherry tomatoes or sliced raw red peppers, carrots or cucumbers

▸ 1 cereal bar (check the fat and sugar content)

▸ 1 apple, orange or banana

Secrets of a successful snacker

Linda Anthony explains her former eating patterns this way: 'I was brought up as an Italian.' Growing up in her family, that meant food, and lots of it. 'We ate when we were happy. We ate when we were sad. We ate when we got together. My whole upbringing revolved around food,' she says. Meals, not snacks, were the focal point – and the meals were huge. 'For lunch, I might have two sandwiches with thick wedges of salami,' she says. 'For dinner, I'd have two or three huge helpings of spaghetti.' She ate mainly at mealtimes but would often continue eating into the night. 'It's embarrassing to say, but I've been known to eat an entire pizza – eight slices – all by myself,' she says.

The results of her poor eating patterns were clear to see. At 1.6m (5ft 3in), she weighed 109kg (17st 2lb), and her blood sugar levels were up to just over 13mmol/l. When it looked as if she might need medication to control her blood glucose levels, an alarm bell went off in her head. 'My mother lost her sight, had kidney trouble, and died from complications of diabetes at the age of 69,' she says. 'It scared me rigid.'

She started a walking programme and began to cut back on her calorie intake at meals. After a lifetime of lavish eating, though, eating less at the table was a tough challenge. That's where having small snacks between meals came in. 'Timing my eating really helped me a lot,' she says. 'I wouldn't feel as hungry when I came to supper, so I would eat less.'

The foods Linda chose made a difference as well. Never a big fruit eater ('My attitude was that it wouldn't stick to your ribs,' she says), she now keeps high-fibre produce such as bananas on hand as a staple. But she loves vegetables, too, and she carries items such as cherry tomatoes with her wherever she goes. 'I even munch on cucumbers,' she says. 'It may not look attractive, but my health is more important to me than worrying about things like that.' Best of all, she has found creative ways to make healthy snacks seem downright sinful. A particular favourite is a chocolate and banana smoothie, made by blending a ripe banana, a tablespoon of cocoa powder, 100ml (3½fl oz) skimmed milk and a scoop of reduced fat vanilla ice cream.

Within six months, she had shed 18kg (2st 12lb). Even more impressive is her long-term progress. After sticking to the plan for 17 months, she lost 54.5kg (8st 8lb) – that's half her starting weight. Her blood sugar now averages about 5mmol/l – well into the normal range. And believe it or not, she says, 'I'm not feeling deprived.'

calories the least, so those you take in are more likely to be stored as fat. In addition, over-eating late in the day makes your body work hard at digestion, hindering the quiet process of tissue repair and muscle building that takes place during sleep – which is important if you are exercising. It can also make you toss and turn in bed, disrupting your sleep and making it even harder to control your blood sugar, as you'll discover in Step Six. Finally, eating into the small hours may contribute to high blood sugar when you wake up in the morning.

Does that mean you have to chew on your fingernails and nothing else while you watch TV in the evening? If you are genuinely hungry, it's fine to have a small snack, but be sure you're not just eating out of habit or because you are bored.

A word about exercise

Is there a best time to exercise? The short answer is yes: any time you can fit it into your schedule. But exercise such as walking and moderate aerobics brings down blood sugar levels both while you do it and for up to a day afterwards. While that is the big payoff, it is also a potential hazard, especially if you are on medication or insulin. If you've just taken oral medication or a dose of insulin to bring down your blood sugar level, then you immediately walk for an hour, the glucose-lowering combination of the treatment and the activity could cause your blood sugar to plummet – a condition known as hypoglycaemia (see page 130).

On the other hand, if you are taking insulin but don't give yourself a large enough dose, your blood sugar may actually rise too high during exercise. That is because when you are physically active, the liver pumps out more glucose, and without adequate insulin your body will have trouble shifting glucose from your blood to working muscles.

Only you and your doctor can sort this out, but you should be able to avoid most problems by following these guidelines.

- Exercise an hour or two after eating. At that point, your blood sugar levels are elevated from food, and you'll have ample glucose to fuel your muscles. At the same time, your digestive system will have finished most of its work, so it won't deplete the energy you need for your workout.

Timing is all

Below is an example of how to achieve well-timed meals and exercise opportunities during the course of a typical day. You should allow an hour (more if possible) between eating and taking exercise.

8am	Breakfast: 3tbsp high-fibre cereal, 200ml (7fl oz) skimmed or semi-skimmed milk, 1 medium banana
9am	Exercise opportunity
10.30am	Snack: 20 red grapes
1pm	Lunch: chicken salad sandwich, a bowl of soup, 1 piece or portion of fresh fruit, a sugar-free drink
2pm	Exercise opportunity
4pm	Snack: 200ml (7fl oz) low-fat, sugar-free yogurt
6.30pm	Evening meal: a small salmon steak (about 125g/4½oz), small jacket potato with 1tbsp low-fat fromage frais, large portion steamed carrots and broccoli, 100g (3½oz) strawberries with 0% fat Greek yogurt
7.30pm	Exercise opportunity
10pm	Snack (optional): 1 oatcake spread with reduced-fat soft cheese

- If you take medication, ask your doctor if you can skip it before exercising or take a lower dose; the drop in blood sugar that occurs during and after physical activity may be able to substitute for the drug. Otherwise, you should avoid exercising when the effects of your medication peak.

- If you use insulin, time your workouts so that you are not active when the effects of the insulin peak – often within the first hour or two after an injection. Your doctor will probably want you to monitor your blood sugar level before and after exercise to see how activity affects it, and based on those results, may want you to adjust your insulin dose before you exercise.

STEP 2 Master the Plate Approach

Now you're ready to get down to the important matter of what to eat. So get a plate and set yourself a place at the table, because your plate, and how you fill it, is the main focus of the 10 Per Cent Plan.

In this step, you'll discover a visual approach to eating that is perfect for people with diabetes. It's called the Plate Approach, and it is amazingly simple.

The Plate Approach rebalances your meals to give you the ideal proportions of vegetables, protein and carbohydrates. It's this perfect balance that will help you to lose weight and keep your blood sugar levels under control. Using the Plate Approach automatically limits your intake of calories – the real goal of any weight-loss plan. It also ensures that you won't get too many carbohydrates at one sitting, with no need for you to keep a tally. Best of all, your plate will contain plenty of food, so you will never feel deprived.

Imagine sitting down to a typical meal – perhaps the one you're having tonight. What do you see? The chances are that meat will dominate the plate. Maybe it's a large steak, gammon steak or pork chop, enough to fill about half the plate. The rest of the plate might contain a large jacket potato with lashings of butter, and maybe, crowded to one side, a few token vegetables – also topped with butter.

A disaster? Pretty much. This is the kind of eating that puts on pounds and clogs arteries. (Remember, heart disease is a serious risk for people with diabetes.) A recent Harvard study of middle-aged and older women even suggests that getting a lot of iron from red meat raises the risk of developing diabetes.

Does that mean you have to give up meat and potatoes? Certainly not. But in order to lose weight and bring down your blood sugar levels you will need to make some adjustments, mostly to the way foods are distributed on your plate. The Plate Approach will help you to do this. It's a simple visual approach to making healthy decisions about what to eat. The biggest change is that the humble helping of vegetables will become a hearty helping, shrinking the space that is left over for fatty meat and starchy carbohydrates – the major sources of calories.

Fighting disease while you fight diabetes

Many low-carbohydrate diets contain few vegetables. Yet vegetables are a rich source of phytochemicals, natural plant chemicals that help the body to defend itself against disease and the ravages of ageing. Broccoli, cabbage and other members of the cruciferous vegetable family help to fight against cancer; tomatoes and red peppers contain lycopene, which also lowers the risk of cancer; carrots are rich in beta-carotene, which helps to protect the eyes; and many vegetables contain bioflavonoids, which help to neutralize unstable molecules called free radicals that can hasten ageing and the development of heart disease and cancer, as well as other chemicals that stimulate the body's immune cells and infection-fighting enzymes.

How the Plate Approach works

Use the three main elements of a typical meal – protein, starch and vegetables – as your starting point. When you dish them out, your plate in effect becomes divided into three sections. Those three sections will be the basis of how you decide what to eat using the Plate Approach. Of course, it's the size of the sections that matters. To picture how your plate should look when you use the Plate Approach, mentally divide it into left and right halves. Then imagine the right half split into two equal parts. Whenever you eat a meal, keep these sections in mind and fill them in the following way.

1. **LEFT SIDE: VEGETABLES** Choose any vegetables you like but remember that potatoes and pulses (see right) do not belong in the vegetable group. For some meals, you can eat fruit instead of (or in addition to) vegetables.

2. **TOP RIGHT: STARCHES** This means carbohydrates such as whole grain bread or pasta, brown rice or potatoes.

3. **BOTTOM RIGHT: PROTEIN FOODS** These include lean red meat, eggs, fish, chicken and turkey, as well as dairy products, such as cheese.

A plate makeover

Using the Plate Approach, the number of calories you save by emphasizing vegetables instead of fatty foods can be significant.

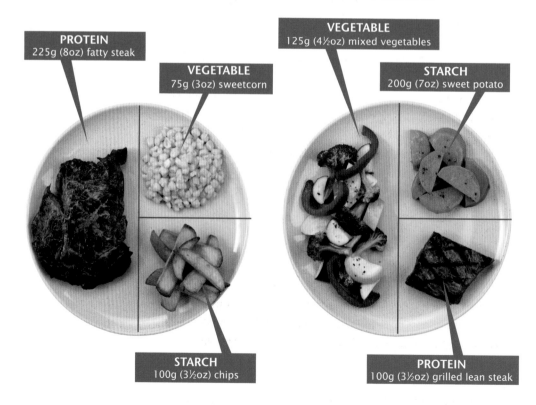

828KCAL

PROTEIN
225g (8oz) fatty steak

VEGETABLE
75g (3oz) sweetcorn

STARCH
100g (3½oz) chips

440KCAL

VEGETABLE
125g (4½oz) mixed vegetables

STARCH
200g (7oz) sweet potato

PROTEIN
100g (3½oz) grilled lean steak

That, in a nutshell, is the Plate Approach. At each meal, feel free to add a drizzle of olive oil or a small amount of margarine or reduced-fat spread. Now eat everything – there's no need to hold back. In fact, you can fill the biggest portion of your plate (the vegetable section) again and again if you still feel hungry. There is *no limit* on the amount of food you can eat from this part of the plate as long as you stop when you feel satisfied. On the right half of the plate, however, you should limit yourself to a single helping of carbohydrate and protein.

Pulses: starch and protein

Pulses (starchy beans) are a special case when it comes to the Plate Approach. The foods in question – such as kidney beans, flageolet beans, cannellini beans, butter beans, black-eyed beans and even baked beans – are all vegetables, but they are packed with plant protein as well as carbohydrates. Because pulses are higher in calories than non-starchy vegetables, you should not eat unlimited amounts, so they don't belong on the vegetable half of your plate. Instead, use them as either a starch or a protein. For example, if you're making chilli, use kidney beans in place of meat to save fat and calories. Or if you want chicken and baked beans for your evening meal, think of the beans as your starch.

Why is the Plate Approach so effective? Partly because it is so intuitive. There are no carbohydrates, or even calories, to count. You don't have to look up any food exchanges or know the Glycaemic Index (GI) values of your favourite foods (see page 64). Eating plenty of vegetables will automatically lower the GI of your meals. And unlike some low-carbohydrate diets, it doesn't require you to virtually eliminate entire food groups. If you find that these other methods work, more power to you, but studies suggest that simpler approaches work just as well while being easier to stick with over the longer term. And of course, it's the long term that counts.

As well as being easy to follow, the Plate Approach has three distinct advantages: it reduces calorie intake, controls carbohydrates and satisfies your hunger.

BENEFIT 1 THE PLATE APPROACH CUTS CALORIES

There's no escaping it: in order to lose weight, you need to take in fewer calories than you burn. The Plate Approach's solution to cutting calorie intake is remarkably simple: eat more vegetables and less of everything else. In the Plate Approach, half of the area on your plate is taken up by vegetables, which are naturally very low in calories, so there is less room available for starches and calorie-dense meats.

Vegetables are low in calories yet high in volume because a lot of their weight comes from water. Such 'high-volume' foods have the advantage of looking big, so they make your brain expect that you will be satisfied by eating them. They also take up more room in your stomach, so they trigger a signal in your brain that makes you stop eating sooner.

By eating more vegetables – raw, steamed or boiled – you automatically eat less fat. That is important, since fat contains more than twice the calories of carbohydrates or protein. Compare the calories in a small amount of cheese with those in a selection of vegetables (below). It's small wonder that researchers in weight-loss programmes, such as one at the University of Alabama in Birmingham, USA, find that when people eat lots of vegetables, their calorie consumption goes down – and they lose weight.

All about calories

For fewer calories than you would get in two small pieces of Cheddar cheese you could fill up on a mountain of vegetables.

210KCAL   **170KCAL**

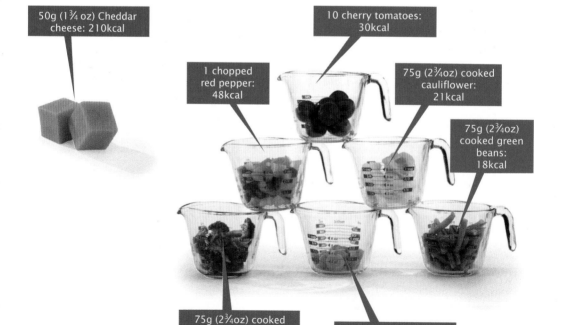

50g (1¾ oz) Cheddar cheese: 210kcal

10 cherry tomatoes: 30kcal

1 chopped red pepper: 48kcal

75g (2¾oz) cooked cauliflower: 21kcal

75g (2¾oz) cooked green beans: 18kcal

75g (2¾oz) cooked broccoli: 18kcal

1 medium raw carrot: 35kcal

Quiz
Making choices, making changes

Succeeding with an eating plan is a combination of habit and knowledge. To find out how close your current eating habits are to the Plate Approach, circle the numbers next to the answers that best reflect your decisions and attitudes.

1. What is the main element of most of your lunches and dinners?
1 Meat
2 Starch (pasta, potatoes, bread, or rice)
3 Vegetables

2. How much room do vegetables usually occupy on your plate?
1 No room – I eat only potatoes
2 About a quarter of the plate
3 Half of the plate or more

3. What is your usual choice when eating bread?
1 White bread
2 Brown bread
3 Wholemeal, granary or multigrain bread

4. Circle all that apply:
1 I tend to eat the same few vegetables all the time
2 Vegetables are boring
3 I would eat more vegetables if I knew how to cook them

5. How often do you eat salads?
1 Only when I go to a restaurant
2 Salads are boring, so I rarely eat them
3 I have a salad with my meals several times a week

6. Which of these fats do you think are good for you?
1 The fats in meat or full-fat dairy products
2 Butter, margarine or vegetable shortening
3 Olive oil, rapeseed oil, or peanut butter

7. How often do you have a low-fat dairy product, such as low-fat or fat-free milk, cheese or yogurt?
1 Rarely or never
2 Once a day
3 Two or three times a day

8. On average, how many soft drinks do you have each day?
1 Three or more
2 One or two
3 None

Add up your score, then turn the page.

Quiz
What your score means

20 to 24 You should have no trouble adjusting to the Plate Approach because you are already applying many of the concepts behind it.

14 to 19 You're making good progress in following the Plate Approach, but you will need to make a few adjustments. Look at the questions you answered with a 3 and ask yourself why these healthy habits seem easier to you than others where you scored lower: there may be lessons you can apply to areas where you need to do more work.

8 to 13 You'll need to start making changes a little at a time to get closer to the Plate Approach. By eating more vegetables and smaller portions of other foods, you will see significant effects on your waistline and blood sugar levels. Focus on questions you answered with a 1 to find out which changes you should focus on.

The logic behind the questions

1. If you answered 'vegetables', you are well on your way to success with the 10 Per Cent Plan. Nothing delivers more nutrients with fewer calories. And you can eat vegetables to your heart's content without worrying about gaining weight. If you answered 'meat' or 'starch', this chapter will show you how to rethink the space that protein and carbohydrate foods occupy on your plate. Adjusting the balance of these foods in your meals will virtually guarantee that you'll lose weight and bring down your blood sugar levels.

2. For most people, potatoes occupy larger areas of the plate than they should. Giving other, non-starchy vegetables a more dominant place on your plate is a sure way to lose weight.

3. If you circled number 3, good for you! Whole-grain bread has less impact on blood sugar than white. 'Brown' bread is not the same as wholemeal or granary bread.

4. If you circled any of these, you are probably stuck in a mental rut when it comes to vegetables. It's time to discover new ways to include more vegetables in your diet.

5. Salads are a perfect way to add vegetables to meals, but if you order a salad in a restaurant, ask for the dressing to be served on the side. Bags of pre-dressed salads make preparation very easy. If you find salads boring, turn to page 71 for some fun topping ideas.

6. Olive and rapeseed oil consist mostly of 'healthy' fats, the kinds that help to stave off heart disease (as opposed to those that contribute to heart disease).

7. You need to have dairy products two or three times a day on the 10 Per Cent Plan, because they are a good source of protein and most products made from milk contain calcium, which can help you to lose weight.

8. Soft drinks add calories without filling you up the way solid foods do. Diet soft drinks are fine – but in moderation, since they tend to stimulate your sweet tooth.

BENEFIT 2 THE PLATE APPROACH CONTROLS CARBOHYDRATES

Contrary to popular belief, carbohydrates are not dietary villains, even if you have diabetes. In fact they are actually the body's main source of energy. Carbohydrates such as whole grains are a major source of B vitamins, iron and fibre, as well as the trace mineral chromium, which is thought to help cells use insulin. Indeed, studies show that eating whole grains lowers the risk of diabetes as well as that of heart disease and stroke. Carbohydrates are also protein sparing, which means that the body uses them first for energy and leaves protein to be used for body repair and other important functions. So they are an essential part of a balanced diet.

Yet because carbohydrates break down into glucose more easily than either fat or protein they have more impact on your blood glucose levels. For example, a big bowl of spaghetti can make your blood sugar soar. So avoid too many carbohydrates at one sitting. The Plate Approach confines starches to one-quarter of your plate, so that you get the right amount. But just as important as limiting your carbohydrate intake is choosing the right ones – the slow-burning type, often known as low GI carbohydrates (see page 64). Examples of these include pasta made from durum wheat, pulses (lentils and beans) and multigrain bread.

Fibre: a side benefit

An extra benefit of the Plate Approach is that your diet will include plenty of fibre from all the vegetables and 'slow-burning' carbohydrates you'll eat. Although not technically a nutrient, since your body can't digest it, fibre has several benefits.

- It slows digestion and keeps blood sugar from rising quickly after a meal. This effect is so powerful that it can lower your overall blood sugar levels. Because it slows digestion, fibre also keeps you feeling full for longer.
- It adds bulk to food, so it makes you feel full without adding calories. One study found that over the course of 10 years, people who ate a lot of high-fibre foods weighed an average of 4.5kg (10lb) less than people who ate little fibre.
- Soluble fibre, found in foods such as beans, barley and oats, can lower your cholesterol levels and reduce your risk of heart disease.
- A high-fibre diet helps to keep you 'regular', making problems such as constipation, Irritable Bowel Syndrome and haemorrhoids (common in people with Type 2 diabetes) less likely. It may also reduce your risk of colon cancer.

BENEFIT 3 THE PLATE APPROACH KEEPS HUNGER IN CHECK

It is important that you include protein at every meal because protein makes you feel full for longer than carbohydrates do. That's remarkable because protein has the same number of calories (4 per gram) as carbohydrates. Protein has the added advantage of being digested more slowly than carbohydrates, so it has a less dramatic impact on your blood sugar level. Beyond these advantages, your body needs protein to build everything from muscles to hardworking enzymes, immune system cells and hormones.

If protein is so great, shouldn't you eat a high-protein diet to lose weight even faster? No. One reason not to include too much protein in your diet is that the high-protein foods we eat most often – especially meat – also tend to be high in saturated fat. That is the type of fat people with diabetes need to eat less of, since it clogs arteries that are already vulnerable to heart disease and makes cells more resistant to insulin (the real problem behind Type 2 diabetes).

Another reason is that filling up on protein would mean eating fewer carbohydrates, the body's primary source of fuel. That would be like ripping the timber out of the walls of your house to feed your boiler instead of using gas or oil. Protein

The Glycaemic Index

The Glycaemic Index (GI) ranks carbohydrate foods according to their effect on blood glucose levels. The faster a food is broken down during digestion, the quicker the rise in blood glucose levels. Foods that cause a rapid rise in blood glucose have a higher GI rating; those that are digested slowly are low on the GI index. But foods with a high GI are not necessarily bad foods, nor are all lower GI foods necessarily healthy.

Extensive research has shown that eating more lower GI carbohydrates can help to control blood glucose levels in diabetes. However, you don't need to know the GI value of everything you're eating, since this can be complex. Instead experts suggest that you follow these simple guidelines to lower the GI of your meals:
- Buy more natural foods rather than processed foods
- Eat wholegrain breakfast cereals such as porridge or muesli
- Choose seeded or grainy breads rather than white or wholemeal bread
- Choose whole fruits rather than fruit juice
- Eat lots of vegetables including plenty of pulses and salads
- Choose pasta and noodles (both low GI) over rice and potatoes (medium/high GI)

doesn't burn as efficiently as carbohydrate or fat. In fact, to be used as fuel, it must undergo chemical changes that release toxic by-products. The body flushes out these toxins in urine, which helps explain why high-protein diets can make you lose weight fast: they cause water loss. When you start to eat a healthy balanced diet again, the weight comes back.

High-protein diets may even endanger your health by over-working your kidneys, and people with diabetes already have an increased risk of kidney damage.

Using the Plate Approach

Now it's time to put the Plate Approach to work. The first step is to make sure your plate is the right size. No, we're not going to ask you to eat your evening meal from a salad plate. Remember, the meals you eat using the Plate Approach are supposed to be generous and satisfying. That means you'll be filling up a standard-size plate, with an eating surface diameter of 40-44cm (8-9in). Don't worry if the lip of the plate makes the dimensions bigger than that: you're only concerned with the area that you actually fill with food. For a ready-made, pre-portioned dish that can help you to use the Plate Approach, you could try using a segmented plate such as those that parents use to serve children.

Not every meal will fit precisely into segments of a plate in the way we have suggested. For example, a stir-fry might have all the right elements – carbohydrate (brown rice), lean protein (chicken strips) and plenty of vegetables (carrots, broccoli and mange tout peas) – but they are all mixed together. That's fine. Once you have grasped the idea of the Plate Approach and get used to seeing how much food goes into each section of the plate, you won't need the divisions to guide you. As long as the bulk of the dish is vegetables, with smaller amounts of rice and poultry, a stir-fry is a perfect Plate Approach meal.

A word about breakfast. We won't ask you to fill half your plate with vegetables at this meal, since few of us eat vegetables in the morning (although if you're making an omelette, fill it with as much produce as possible). Instead, substitute fruit – blueberries, strawberries or a banana – or unsweetened orange juice for vegetables.

In Step Three, we will show you options for every meal so that you can see how easy it is to make the Plate Approach work over the course of a week.

Filling the vegetable side of the plate

Almost all vegetables are on the approved list for unlimited eating with the Plate Approach. The exceptions are potatoes and pulses such as kidney and cannellini beans (see page 59). Because these starchy vegetables are higher in calories than other vegetables, they belong in the smaller starch section of your plate, and you're limited to one serving of these.

Many of us have a tendency to lump all vegetables together as if they were a single food. But vegetables can be sweet, bitter or bland; big or small; and green, yellow, orange, red, brown and every shade in between. Given the sheer bounty of natural foods at your disposal, how do you decide which to eat?

The first thing to do is to vote with your taste buds and eat the produce you like. But if you tend to eat only one vegetable, such as green beans, try to vary your dietary routine. This will help to ensure that you get all the nutrients you need. A serving of broccoli, for example, contains several important nutrients, but not necessarily the same ones as a serving of asparagus. Varying the vegetables you eat can also help you to lose weight. Studies suggest that people

Help!

My family hates vegetables, and I'm not willing to make separate meals. How do I get round this problem?

The first thing to do is explore why they don't like vegetables. The problem could be a simple matter of preparation. If you have always cooked vegetables, maybe your family would like them better raw – or vice-versa. It's a common error to overcook vegetables, making them mushy and bland. Instead, try lightly steaming vegetables such as cauliflower so they're appealingly hot but still have a gratifying crunch. Or maybe your family would be more open to veggies if they were incorporated into casseroles or stir-fries rather than served as a side dish.

Also, don't assume that past dislikes are set in stone. Tastes change with age, and you may well find that family members will now eat foods they once wouldn't touch. What's more, studies show that if people are exposed to a food more frequently they are more likely to accept it. So keep trying. And don't forget: you have diabetes, and good food is good medicine. Maybe your family members are the ones who need to adapt.

who eat a variety of foods, especially vegetables, tend to consume less fat and are less likely to be overweight than people who have become stuck in dietary ruts.

Start by first choosing vegetables with star nutritional power. As a rule of thumb, vivid colours – dark greens and bright reds or yellows – signal that a vegetable is packed with vitamins, minerals and other vital nutrients. You can't go wrong with the following.

Asparagus

A 75g (3oz) portion of steamed asparagus contains only 20kcal, but plenty of vitamin C, folate, B vitamins and good amounts of fibre.

TIP Use asparagus spears within two days of purchase because they lose their vitamin C quickly. Steam the spears and then sprinkle with lemon juice or low-sodium soy sauce

Vegetables provide volume

Vegetables add volume to your meals without adding lots of calories. Bulking up dishes such as pasta with steamed vegetables instead of high-fat sauce allows you to eat significantly more for the same number of calories.

380KCAL

380KCAL

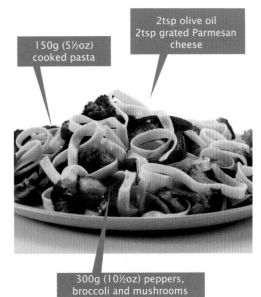

150g (5½oz) cooked pasta

150g (5½oz) cooked pasta

2tsp olive oil
2tsp grated Parmesan cheese

125ml (4fl oz) cheese sauce

300g (10½oz) peppers, broccoli and mushrooms

or a sprinkling of lemon zest for extra flavour. Or try roasting them in the oven with a little olive oil. You could make instant asparagus soup by puréeing cooked asparagus, heating it with a little milk and adding chopped parsley or tarragon.

Peppers

Whether red, yellow or green, peppers are full of B vitamins and vitamin C. Red peppers also contain beta-carotene, which the body converts to beta-carotene, a nutrient that helps to protect the eyes.

TIP With their large lobes and airy interiors, peppers are perfect for stuffing, but first remove the seeds, which can be bitter. Use a sharp knife to cut a circle around the stem, then lift it out, along with the interior membranes that hold the seeds. Rinse out any stragglers that are left inside the pepper.

Broccoli

This cruciferous vegetable is often referred to as the king of vegetables. It is packed with vitamins A and C as well as other antioxidants (compounds that help to guard against cancer and heart disease, among other things), and it even contains calcium, which may help to lower high blood pressure (common in people with Type 2 diabetes).

TIP Overcooking can degrade some of broccoli's nutrients, so steam florets lightly, or quickly stir-fry them in a little olive oil. To eat them almost raw but cooked just enough to soften them, blanch the spears in boiling water for about 3 minutes.

Vegetable seasoning guide

Asparagus	Lemon, garlic, oregano
Aubergine	Basil, garlic, crushed tomato
Broccoli	Garlic, soy sauce, mustard, dark sesame oil
Carrots	Lemon, orange, curry powder, ginger, dill, raspberry vinegar
Cauliflower	Basil, curry powder
Green beans	Garlic, soy sauce, sesame seeds
Mushrooms	Parsley, thyme, spring onions, chives, sherry, balsamic vinegar
Peas	Mint, garlic
Spinach	Garlic, soy sauce, sea salt, nutmeg, balsamic vinegar
Squash/pumpkin	Lemon, rosemary, tomato, garlic, basil
Tomato	Basil, garlic, oregano, balsamic vinegar, Parmesan cheese

Brussels sprouts

These little cabbage-like nodes are rich in vitamin C. They are also an excellent source of lutein, an antioxidant that may reduce the risk of developing cataracts – a serious concern when you are already at increased risk of eye damage due to diabetes.

TIP The stems are tougher than the leaves, so cut an 'X' across the base of each sprout before steaming to allow heat inside the core to soften it. The sprouts will cook evenly for consistent tenderness. For the mildest taste, choose frozen baby Brussels sprouts. For the best flavour, cook them lightly so they're still a little crisp.

Cauliflower

The densely packed florets of a cauliflower head are a great source of B vitamins, which help the body to metabolize glucose.

TIP Although some recipes call for serving a head of cooked cauliflower intact, when it is broken or cut into florets it cooks more quickly, so more nutrients are preserved. Faster cooking also holds back cauliflower's pungent odour, which intensifies the longer you heat it.

Dark, leafy greens

Greens such as spinach, Swiss chard, bok choy and winter cabbage are some of the few plant sources of zinc, a mineral that protects insulin-producing beta cells in the pancreas. Zinc is lost in the urine when blood sugar is too high. These leafy greens are also useful sources of calcium and magnesium – minerals that have been shown to decrease the risk of diabetes – as well as containing antioxidants that help to protect your eyes and combat heart disease.

Instant vegetables five easy ways

Introducing more vegetables into your diet doesn't have to involve time-consuming preparation, especially if you start with these five 'convenience' foods.

Canned tomatoes These are endlessly useful as an ingredient in sauces and casseroles, not to mention chilli.

Frozen stir-fry vegetables Add them to pasta, stir-fries, casseroles or soup, or top them with low-fat grated cheese.

Frozen spinach Add it to cheese pizza, pasta sauce or omelettes; or use in frittata.

Bags of salad Use as the base for a super-fast lunch or light meal by adding beans, vegetables, canned tuna – anything you want. Include salad in sandwiches.

Canned sweetcorn and beans Choose those without added sugar or salt, or rinse well before using in casseroles or salads.

TIP Spinach leaves tend to attract grit. Before cooking or serving, place them in a bowl or sink of cool water. Swish them gently to remove the grit, then drain and repeat if necessary. To dry the leaves, give them a whirl in a salad spinner.

IT'S ALL IN THE PREPARATION

Almost all vegetables are inherently good for you, but beware of transforming low-calorie vegetables into high-calorie ones by frying them in oil or smothering them with toppings, such as cheese sauces, full-fat salad dressings or butter. By adding just 1 teaspoon of butter, you more than double or triple the calories in a serving of vegetables.

This doesn't mean that you have to resign yourself to bland and tasteless vegetables. There are plenty of ways you can add flavour to them without adding excess calories.

ROAST Roasting vegetables brings out delicious sweetness. Aubergines, onions, red peppers, courgettes, mushrooms and carrots are all perfect candidates. Simply slice them, brush with a little olive oil or Italian dressing, and roast at 200°C (400°F, Gas mark 6) until done.

SEASON Think beyond butter when it comes to seasoning vegetables. Try lemon juice, garlic salt or herbs. Balsamic or white wine vinegar also gives an appealing tang to spinach and other greens.

TOP Add low-fat grated cheese or Parmesan, toasted sliced almonds, sesame seeds or walnuts.

ADOPT A LOW-EFFORT APPROACH

Why don't vegetables play a greater role in the British diet, as they do in some other countries? One answer may be that preparing vegetables can often seem labour intensive. But vegetables don't always have to be served as sensational side dishes or main courses. Here are nine simple ways in which to introduce more vegetables into your meals or boost their plate appeal.

1. Stock your larder and freezer with canned and frozen vegetables. They can be as nutritious as fresh vegetables because they are picked at their peak, when they are at their most nutrient-rich. Frozen vegetables are flash-frozen,

which seals in the nutrients until the vegetables are thawed. Don't worry about canned vegetables losing nutrients that leach into water in cans. The amounts are small, and you lose nothing if you use the water in dishes such as soup.

2. Add some canned or frozen vegetables, such as carrots, peas, chopped spinach or beans, to every soup you make.

3. Dress up a cheese pizza with mushrooms, peppers, spinach and broccoli.

4. For an instant, perfectly dressed salad, open a bag of pre-washed salad or mixed greens. Add a tablespoon of olive oil and a splash of lemon juice or balsamic vinegar, and shake.

5. Stock your kitchen or larder with vegetables that keep well, such as carrots, celery, onions, cucumbers, squash and garlic. That way, you will always have produce on hand even when you are unable to shop for more perishable items.

Making salads interesting

Plain lettuce salads are boring – no wonder some people think they don't like salad! To add greater appeal, vary the greens, and choose two or three of these items as toppings.

- Almonds
- Artichoke hearts
- Baby corn
- Chickpeas
- Raisins
- Grapefruit sections
- Hearts of palm
- Kidney beans
- Linseeds
- Mandarin orange wedges

- Mango slices
- Olives
- Peanuts
- Pecans
- Raspberries
- Red grapes
- Starfruit slices
- Strawberry slices
- Sunflower seeds
- Walnuts
- Water chestnuts

6. To save time, buy pre-cut vegetables.

7. Put raw vegetables out on a plate while you're making your evening meal so you can snack on them instead of higher-calorie temptations such as crisps or other starchy foods. Find a low-fat vegetable dip which the whole family enjoys to go with the crudités.

8. Lightly steam vegetables in a steamer for 3 to 5 minutes, until the colour turns brighter (this is the point at which they are most nutritious). Then eat the crisp-tender vegetables either hot with the meal or cold as a snack.

9. Add frozen stir-fry vegetables to canned chicken soup and heat for about 5 minutes for a quick, nutritious soup. Add soy sauce or miso paste for an Asian flavour.

LEARNING TO LIKE VEGETABLES

What if you simply don't like the taste of vegetables? If that's the case, it is probably because you are not accustomed to eating them. People who think they don't like vegetables can actually end up loving them if they introduce them gradually, giving the palate a chance to develop a taste for them. The following strategies will also help.

- Try preparing vegetables in different ways, since texture, not taste, may be the problem. Cooking them a little less or more than usual will change the texture and perhaps even the taste. You may also find that you like some vegetables better raw than cooked.

- Serve 'baby' versions of vegetables such as carrots, green beans and Brussels sprouts, which tend to have a more appealing texture and a slightly sweeter flavour.

- Disguise your vegetables – for example, in vegetable juice or salsa, which contains onions, tomatoes and peppers. Use salsa as a dip for vegetables or a topping for baked potatoes.

- Add chopped or puréed carrots to cottage pie; this disguises the vegetable without substantially changing the taste of the meat. Similarly, put chopped or puréed spinach (or any other vegetable that appeals to you) into lasagne, bread dough or pasta sauce.

FRUIT: NOT TO BE FORGOTTEN

So far, we have been talking mostly about vegetables, but fruit also deserves a place on your plate. Many people believe that fructose, the sugar that occurs naturally in fruit, makes fruit off-limits for people with diabetes, but that is not the case. People with diabetes can eat any kind of fruit. Fruits, in common with vegetables, are rich in nutrients, low in fat and high in fibre. They are also relatively low in calories compared with many other foods.

At the same time, you can't eat fruit with abandon. Aim to get three or four portions, spaced at intervals throughout the day. As a guide, a portion is: one medium-sized fruit (apple, orange, banana or pear); two smaller fruits (apricots, plums); a large slice of a larger fruit (melon or pineapple); a cupful of strawberries, raspberries or grapes; or 2-3 tablespoons fresh fruit salad. A 150ml (5fl oz) glass of fruit juice also counts as a portion, but you should limit yourself to a maximum of one glass a day of fruit juice as this can cause glucose levels to rise more quickly. Here are some approaches to consider:

- Have one portion of fruit with each meal: berries or melon at breakfast, an apple or banana at lunch, and a fruit-based dessert after dinner.

- Eat fruit at breakfast, then as a snack at mid-morning and mid-afternoon.

- Reserve fruit entirely for snacks at mid-morning, mid-afternoon and bedtime.

As with vegetables, you should eat a variety of fruits every day, since different fruits provide you with different nutrients.

It's also important to ensure that most of your fruit portions are the whole fruit rather than just the juice. Many of the nutrients and much of the fibre found in the skin, flesh and seeds of fruit are eliminated during juicing. In addition, because the fibre from the fruit has been removed and the physical structure of the fruit has been disrupted, fruit juice is digested more quickly than the whole fruit so blood glucose rises more quickly. The juicing process also squashes the natural sugars out of the cells that normally contain them, thereby increasing the GI, and concentrates the calories. What's more, drinking fruit juice doesn't give you the gratifying effort of chewing, so it's easy to take in additional calories without feeling satisfied.

The carbohydrate quarter

When we advised you to fill a quarter of your plate with carbohydrates, the chances are you didn't say, 'Great! I'll fill it with sweets, biscuits and cakes', although you might have done, because those are all carbohydrates. But unlike other carbohydrates, sugary foods contribute very little in the way of nutrition but plenty of calories. And that's not the only issue.

More importantly, especially for people with diabetes, is the way in which different types of carbohydrate are digested. 'Refined' carbohydrates, such as sugar-rich drinks, white bread, cereals made primarily from rice or corn, and most baked goods and snack foods, are easily digested and are generally quickly broken down into glucose, which sends your blood sugar soaring. Your body pumps out more insulin to handle the sudden flood of glucose and, in response to the insulin, blood sugar plummets, leaving you shaky and hungry again in no time. Needless to say, these are not the carbohydrates we want you to focus on.

CHOOSE WHOLE GRAIN, NOT REFINED

The foods that should occupy the quarter of your plate dedicated to carbohydrates are low GI carbohydrates or whole grains that have not been stripped of their fibre and nutrients. These whole grains take longer to digest and therefore will not raise your blood sugar as dramatically as processed carbohydrates do. They also contain far more vitamins and minerals than refined carbohydrates.

Many people in the UK aren't accustomed to eating whole grains and may not know where to begin. Fortunately, it's not difficult.

- Buy bread and rolls which contain whole grains or seeds. You should see the name of the grain as the first ingredient. This is the easiest way to shift the balance from high GI to low GI carbohydrates in your diet. Don't be fooled by words that manufacturers sometimes use to make their products sound healthier than they are. For example, colouring a loaf of bread brown and calling it wheat bread doesn't make it wholemeal. Or saying a product is 'made with wheat flour' could be true of both wholemeal bread and angel cake. If a product is truly wholegrain, the label should list the grain, such as whole oats, as the first ingredient on the label.

- Eat a breakfast of champions. Some of the most accessible (and tasty) sources of whole

---

Five things to do with a bag of barley

Barley is one of the richest dietary sources of cholesterol-lowering soluble fibre, but people don't often think of including it in their diets – and maybe you are not even sure how to. Here are some ideas to get you started.

1. Add it to soups and stews as a more nutritious alternative to pasta or noodles.

2. Make a side dish by sautéing vegetables such as onions, garlic and carrots, then adding barley and herbs, such as sage and thyme, and simmering in water according to the package directions.

3. Try a barley salad topped with a sprinkling of Parmesan cheese.

4. Add barley to chilli as a textured thickener that will allow you to use less meat.

5. Use it in place of rice to stuff peppers.

If you want to lower your blood sugar faster, watch what you drink. Some beverages pack on the pounds, while others can actually help to moderate glucose swings – as can a certain spice that we encourage you to cook with.

Cut down on fizzy drinks

These beverages have no nutritional value, but each 330ml (10fl oz) can of cola or fizzy drink contains 135kcal and the equivalent of 9 teaspoons of sugar. Also, studies show that calories from these drinks don't fill you up the way food does, so you end up consuming more calories throughout the day than you would if you derived those calories from something solid.

If you usually drink three cans of cola a day – not unusual if you drink it more out of habit or convenience than desire – you can easily cut an impressive 450kcal by switching to another beverage, such as:

- Water. It contains no calories and quenches thirst better than sugary drinks. Choose plain water or fruit-flavoured varieties, but choose sugar-free brands of flavoured water as some brands contain as many calories as soft drinks. Check the label if in doubt.

- Diet drinks with noncaloric sweeteners.

- Lemonade. Making your own with fresh lemon juice and sweetening it with a sugar substitute cuts out the calories, saving more than 100kcal compared with shop-bought lemonade.

Enjoy a good cup of tea

If you're a tea drinker, try green tea. Compounds called polyphenols in green tea also appear to help fight against diabetes. In one recent study, cells from diabetic rats that drank green tea soaked up twice as much blood sugar as cells from rats that drank plain water. Drinking black tea had no effect on blood sugar absorption.

Merit in moderation

Unless your GP has told you to avoid alcohol for a specific medical reason, you can feel free to enjoy the occasional glass of wine or beer. In fact alcohol in moderation may even help prevent cardiovascular problems associated with diabetes. But you should adhere to safe drinking limits. The guidelines for people with diabetes are 21 units a week for men and 14 units a week for women. Be aware that alcohol lowers blood glucose levels so don't drink when your blood glucose is low. It is also high in calories so if you're trying to lose weight don't drink more than seven units of alcohol a week.

Spice it up

Add a dash of cinnamon to your food whenever you get a chance. Recent research shows that the spice lowers blood sugar by boosting the activity of insulin. As little as ½ teaspoon a day can lower blood sugar by as much as 29 per cent.

Use cinnamon to flavour chicken stew or sprinkle it on puddings such as apple pie (you'll find a low-fat recipe on page 125). Or brew up a pot of cinnamon tea. Simply boil 4 cups of water, add four cinnamon sticks, and simmer for 20 minutes. Strain before drinking.

grains can be found in cereals such as porridge, muesli or Kashi. Read the labels and look for a cereal that contains at least 3g of fibre per serving – the higher the fibre content, the better.

- Give a boost to homemade baked goods by replacing one-third of the white flour with wholemeal flour.

- Use whole wheat pasta, preferably made with durum wheat. It is becoming more widely available, along with whole wheat couscous, bulgur and other whole grain products.

- Switch to brown rice. It may take a little while to get used to it if you are accustomed to eating white rice, but soon you will find yourself enjoying its somewhat nutty taste and slightly crunchy texture.

Help!

I'm addicted to carbohydrates. How can I overcome my cravings?

Some people have a strong urge to eat – and often overeat – pasta and bread as well as biscuits and chocolate. Don't blame yourself for lack of willpower, though. There may in fact be a physical reason you crave starches. They raise blood levels of the amino acid tryptophan, which increases production of the feel-good hormone serotonin. Some experts believe that people who crave carbohydrates actually have a faulty serotonin feedback mechanism. Whether or not that is true, you're not a slave to brain chemistry. Here are some ways to calm your cravings.

- Fix the mood, not the food. Going outside for some fresh air, visiting a friend, holding a baby, playing with a pet, exercising or enjoying a hobby can all distract you, lift your mood, keep you out of the kitchen, and help to chase away cravings.

- Limit the damage. If chocolate is your weakness, keep it in the freezer: it's more difficult to wolf down when it's frozen solid. Better still, don't keep it in the house.

- Fight food with food. When you're driven to eat salty carbohydrates, try getting more calcium from dairy foods or other sources. Studies have found that people with low intakes of this mineral are more prone to salt cravings.

- Give yourself a 'fix' of your trigger food every day. If you deny yourself altogether, you may simply end up wanting the food more. Eating a moderate amount daily should stave off cravings.

- In some cases, cutting out sugary foods such as chocolate and biscuits completely for two weeks makes the cravings for those foods virtually disappear. Try it!

- Food cravings sometimes indicate a need for fluids. Drink a large glass of water, then wait 10 minutes or so and see if the craving passes.

BE SMART ABOUT SWEET FOODS

Do desserts have a place in your diet when you have diabetes? The answer is a qualified yes. You can eat any type of food as long as you keep calories under control. Forget the old notion that sugar is bad for you. Sugar is just another form of carbohydrate, and it is now known that, generally speaking, sugar does not raise the blood glucose level any higher than other carbohydrates. According to Diabetes UK, sugar can be eaten by people with diabetes who are not overweight provided that it is used in the context of a healthy diet and does not account for more than 10 per cent of the calories obtained from carbohydrates. Sugary snacks and desserts can raise blood sugar faster than other foods because they are virtually fibre-free – and fibre slows digestion of food thereby taming its impact on blood sugar.

Sugar contains calories but has virtually no nutrients. To avoid taking in extra calories while still indulging your sweet tooth, use 'intense' or 'sugar-free' sweeteners which do not affect blood glucose levels. Although the safety of artificial sweeteners has been questioned, numerous studies have shown them to be safe in the quantities normally used in food and the Food Standards Agency states that they are thoroughly tested for safety before they are permitted for use. The following sugar substitutes are widely available.

ASPARTAME Sold under brand names such as NutraSweet and Canderel, aspartame is 200 times sweeter than sugar. It is used as a sugar substitute and to sweeten foods or drinks that are not cooked, because it can break down and lose its sweetness when heated.

ACESULFAME-K About as sweet as aspartame but stable when heated, acesulfame-K is found in sweet foods that you cook (gelatins, puddings), beverages and chewing gum. It is also used as a sugar substitute.

SACCHARIN Primarily used in processed foods, saccharin is also available as a sugar substitute under brand names such as Sweet N' Low.

SUCRALOSE Although it is made from sugar, sucralose (Splenda) is chemically altered so the body does not recognize it as a carbohydrate and doesn't absorb it. Used in a variety of low-calorie foods and drinks and as a sugar substitute, it is heat stable, so you can cook with it.

Choosing the right protein

How do you fill the protein corner of your plate? Unless you are a vegetarian (in which case protein is found in pulses such as kidney beans, black-eyed beans and lentils), your answer is probably 'with meat'. And meat has its role to play in the 10 Per Cent Plan – as long as you choose carefully.

Meat contains fat, which is a drawback because fat means calories. We don't propose that you should eliminate fat from your diet – that wouldn't make sense. Fat adds flavour, richness and texture to foods. It makes you feel full and satisfied. And it helps the body absorb fat-soluble vitamins such as vitamins A and E. In fact, people who cut out too much fat from their diets are less likely to succeed at losing weight. That doesn't mean, though, that you can eat all the fat you want or that every type of fat is good for you. In Step Three, we will show you how you can put together meals that provide a good helping of protein based on the following guidelines.

CUT BACK ON SATURATED FAT

The culprit in most heart problems that are blamed on fat intake is saturated fat, the type found in meat and full-fat dairy products such as cheese. Saturated fat raises 'bad' LDL cholesterol, the kind that clogs blood vessels and can lead to heart attacks and strokes – and you already have an increased risk of these when you have diabetes. Just as important for you, research shows that saturated fat may increase insulin resistance and make blood sugar control more difficult.

Five things you can do with a can of beans

First, drain and rinse the beans, then:

1. Add chickpeas or kidney beans to a salad for a filling fix of protein.
2. Pour canned beans into soup or chilli.
3. Add some to pasta sauce for an Italian-style dish.
4. Make a tasty black bean and sweetcorn salad (see recipe on page 233).
5. Mash kidney beans or black beans and serve on tortillas.

The trick is to choose lean meats and low-fat dairy products. It's no great hardship: in the next chapter you'll find plenty of meals that fit the bill. Even some of your favourite unhealthy foods – such as burgers, macaroni cheese and fried chicken – get the lower-fat treatment in the recipes beginning on pages 108-127.

In general, you should:

- Choose meats that are relatively low in saturated fats. Before cooking, trim off any visible fat from steaks, chops and cutlets, and from cubes of meat that are to be used in casseroles or stews. (Put meat in the freezer 20 minutes beforehand and it will firm it up, making it easier to cut.)

- Cook casseroles and stews ahead of time and allow them to cool overnight in the fridge. A layer of congealed fat will form on the top which can easily be skimmed off. Or drop a few ice cubes into a warm casserole or stew: the fat will solidify around them and they can then be lifted out.

- Eat chicken without the skin. (You can leave the skin on while cooking to help keep the meat moist, then remove it before eating.)

- Choose lower-fat versions of dairy foods. Skimmed milk, for example, is virtually fat-free, while whole milk gets almost half of its fat calories from saturated fat. For 100kcal, you can have either 300ml (10fl oz) skimmed milk or 150ml (5fl oz) whole milk.

FAVOUR OILS, NUTS AND FISH

Not all fat is bad for your heart or your insulin sensitivity (although all fat is high in calories). In fact, some fat – the unsaturated kind – is actually good for you. This type of fat lowers your 'bad' cholesterol rather than raising it. And one type of unsaturated fat, called monounsaturated fat, has even been shown to help reduce insulin resistance and make blood sugar easier to control. Sources of monounsaturated fat are:

- Almonds and other nuts
- Avocados
- Olive and rapeseed oil
- Peanuts and peanut butter
- Seeds

However, you'll still have to watch how much you eat, because at 9 kilocalories per gram, even 'good' fat can pack on the pounds. For example, peanut butter makes an excellent protein choice for a quick lunch or snacks, but you should limit yourself to 2 tablespoons because of its high fat content.

Fatty fish are another source of 'good' fats: omega-3 fatty acids. These fats are the kind proven to cut the risk of a fatal heart attack – so people with diabetes should eat them. Omega-3 fatty acids are found in:

- Oily, cold-water fish such as salmon, tuna, canned sardines, and mackerel. Using the Plate Approach, you should aim to fill the protein quarter of your plate with fish two or three times a week.

- Shellfish such as prawns, lobster and mussels. They contain smaller amounts of omega-3s but are low in saturated fat and calories. They also contain other important nutrients for people with diabetes, including vitamin B_{12} and zinc.

- Certain vegetable oils such as linseed, walnut and rapeseed. But recent evidence suggests that these may not bestow the same benefits as oily fish.

KEEP DAIRY FOODS ON THE MENU

Dairy deserves a special mention because foods such as low-fat cheese and fat-free milk and yogurt are high in both protein and calcium. Why is calcium important? Studies have found that if you get adequate amounts of calcium this can help you to lose weight. This is because a lack of adequate calcium triggers the release of a hormone called calcitriol, which prompts the body to store fat. Eating two or three servings of calcium-rich dairy foods per day helps to keep calcitriol levels low so your body burns more fat and stores less. Taking calcium supplements doesn't seem to produce the same effect, which has led researchers to conclude that dairy foods may have some other, as-yet-undiscovered, weight-loss advantage as well.

Not everyone tolerates the lactose in milk well, but if you are bothered by symptoms such as bloating and gas, you can ease dairy into your diet by having small amounts with meals, which slows the rate at which lactose enters your system. You can also forgo milk in favour of dairy foods that are naturally lower in lactose, such as low-fat cheese and yogurt.

Succeeding with soul food

Shirley Smith already loved vegetables when she joined the DO IT study – but that wasn't helping her to lose weight or control her diabetes. 'I like my greens in the traditional African style,' she says, 'just the way my mother made them – cooked with fatty ham hocks or salt pork.' These fat-laden cooking techniques and a love of fried chicken (especially dark meat, the fattiest kind), bread rolls and desserts such as sweet potato pie boosted her weight to 99kg (15st 8lb) and her blood sugar levels into the region of 10.8mmol/l.

The Plate Approach helped Shirley, an assistant professor of nursing, to rethink her meals, starting with smaller portions in the carbohydrate and protein quarters. 'I cut back on meat and bread rolls quite a bit,' she says. 'Eating chicken at home, I'd normally have the leg and thigh, but now I just have one piece. And if I'm served chicken breast at a conference, I'll only eat half of it, skip the roll, and eat all of the salad.'

Eating fewer carbohydrates and less protein automatically left more room for vegetables – but she also needed to change the way she cooked her vegetables. Her solution was to replace high-fat meats such as ham hocks with smoked turkey parts. 'I simmer the turkey in water on low for, oh, probably 45 minutes, then I put in the greens and cook slowly for hours, the way my mother showed me,' she says. 'I add celery and onions to make it more tasty. It's very good.' Just as important, she started eating more salads and fruit, which she always liked but wasn't accustomed to eating. Now, she typically eats two servings of vegetables with lunch and dinner, so they make up about half the amount of food in her meals.

By taking these steps (along with getting regular exercise and not skipping breakfast), Shirley lost 16 per cent of her body weight and her blood sugar levels dropped well into the normal range of about 5.2mmol/l. Understanding that no food is completely off-limits, she still sometimes cooks her greens the traditional way, 'but I save that for special occasions such as Christmas,' she says, 'and then I'll eat less pie.' Although her weight and blood sugar have fluctuated with stress and age (she is 68), she has kept both below what they were when she started the plan three years ago. 'The plan taught me a lot about how to eat, especially what an impact eating lots of fruits and vegetables can have,' she says. 'And I found that it works.'

STEP 3 Master your portions

The Plate Approach reduces calorie intake simply and significantly by confining higher-calorie foods such as meat and starches to half of your plate. But how high should you heap those potatoes, and just how big is a proper portion of beef or chicken? What if you're not dining on a plate at all? Can the breakfast muffin you eat on a napkin or the sandwich you pack for lunch be as large as you like? Not exactly.

This chapter will help you to master portion sizes – and implement the Plate Approach – by showing you a generous sampling of real-life, easy-to-make meals.

These breakfasts, lunches and dinners represent the perfect balance of vegetables (or fruit), carbohydrates and protein, all in proper portion sizes. We even give you healthy, low-calorie snacks, desserts and menus for special occasions, tailor-made for people with diabetes. These meals prove that eating well doesn't mean that you have to enjoy your food any less.

You know by now that if you want to lose weight and bring down your blood sugar, you have to pay attention to what you eat. But what about *how much* you eat? It's not a point you can afford to ignore, although most people underestimate its importance. In one recent US survey, 78 per cent of people said that eating certain types of food was more important for losing weight than reducing calorie intake. It's little wonder that so many of us are still trying to shed weight.

In case we haven't said it enough, we'll say it again. The key to losing weight is eating fewer calories (and burning more calories through exercise). The Plate Approach builds in calorie control by assigning carbohydrates and protein – which provide most of our calories – to their quarter-plate positions. But it still helps to have a grasp of what an appropriate serving size is.

Working out how much food to buy and cook so that your plate is divided as it should be takes a little practice. Use the chart on page 85 to help you, and keep referring to it for as long as you need to. Eventually, serving and eating food in these portions will become second nature.

Perfect portions all day, every day

BREAKFAST

Breakfast is the most important meal of your day. You should aim for an intake of about 350kcal – and don't shy away from a healthy cooked breakfast. Remember that consuming more calories in the morning can help you to eat less later on in the day.

One challenge with breakfast is getting protein into your meal. The breakfasts on the following pages all provide you with the protein you need, even when you're not sitting down to an omelette. Milk, yogurt and peanut butter fit the bill. (For the fastest possible complete breakfast, simply grab a pot of fat-free, sugar-free fruit yogurt and top it with 3 to 4 tablespoons of high-fibre cereal.)

A word about fruit juice: limit yourself to drinking no more than 175ml (6fl oz). Although it does contain important nutrients, juice is a concentrated source of calories, and it lacks the fibre that makes fresh fruit filling. All that natural sugar with little fibre to slow its digestion also means that fruit juice may send your blood sugar level soaring.

Finally, if you'd rather opt for cereal than the breakfasts here, choose a brand that contains at least 3g of fibre per serving. Top it with fruit for a perfect Plate Approach meal.

LUNCH

What makes a perfect lunch? For a start, eating it a maximum of five hours after breakfast (and preferably sooner). You also want a meal that will energize you rather than send you into an afternoon slump. That means one with ample protein but little fat. The lunches on the following pages provide a healthy balance of nutrients and are easy to prepare.

You probably have a little more time for lunch than for breakfast, so don't rush. Slowly savouring your food will make you feel more satisfied, so you will be less likely to overeat.

To ensure that you get plenty of vegetables, add a salad, or fill up your sandwich with lettuce and tomato or cucumbers, bean sprouts, onions or roasted red peppers from a jar. A piece of fruit is the simplest dessert.

DINNER

Most people think of dinner as the main meal of the day, but the feasts we have come up with are designed (for the most part) to provide no more calories than the meals you eat for lunch. In fact, you can think of these as lunch previews, since all of them are perfect for reheating and eating as leftovers another day. Remember that you should finish eating dinner at least four hours before bedtime to give your body time to digest your meal and use up most of those calories before your metabolism slows down for the night. Some of our fastest meals involve little more than assembling ingredients. In general, if you need to prepare dinner in a hurry, start with a bag of frozen stir-fry vegetables and go from there.

SNACKS

Healthy snacks can demand some advance planning because vending machines offer a limited range of options. In fact, it's not a bad idea to abandon the whole concept of 'snack foods',

A visual guide to portion sizes

FOOD ITEM	AMOUNT	PICTURE IT AS
Meat	75g (3oz)	A piece the size of a pack of cards
Fish	75g (3oz)	A piece the size of a cheque book
Cooked pasta, rice or noodles	2 heaped tbsp	A pile the size of a computer mouse
Bread roll	1 medium	About the size of a tennis ball
Potatoes	1 medium	About the size of a light bulb
Breakfast cereal	25g (1oz)	A medium-sized bowl
Low-fat cheese	40g (1½oz)	A piece the size of a small matchbox
Low-fat yogurt	200ml (7fl oz)	About the size of a takeaway coffee cup
Butter	1 knob	A cube the size of a dice
Vegetables or fruit	75g (3oz)	A pile the size of a cricket ball (you are in fact permitted to eat an unlimited amount of vegetables)

which typically includes crisps, biscuits and chocolate. What does that leave? Plenty. Reach into your refrigerator or larder for small helpings of foods that are staples of regular meals, such as vegetables, fruit, yogurt and cereal. Then branch out to nuts or dried fruit. The snacks on the following pages make great hunger stoppers that are easy to carry with you or stash in a cool bag or small office fridge and contain 150kcal or less. Another option if you're near a microwave is a cup of any soup that isn't cream based.

Remember, on the 10 Per Cent Plan, we *want* you to snack once or twice a day. Snacking is a great way to keep hunger and blood sugar under control and help you to lose weight.

MEALS FOR SPECIAL OCCASIONS

There's nothing like a party to encourage over-eating. That's true whenever food is the focal point of socializing, but especially when eating is linked with time-honoured tradition. Fortunately, you don't have to abandon any family rituals to keep calories under control. Watching portion sizes and resisting seconds will help. If you're producing a traditional feast, prepare low-fat foods, such as chicken breast, turkey breast and lean ham, in ways that keep fat to a minimum. Then focus your attention on making healthy choices with side dishes and desserts.

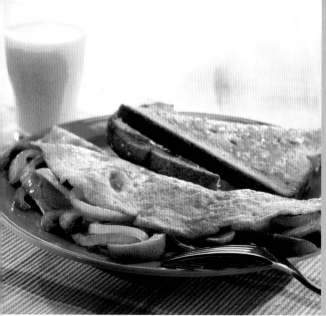

WEEKEND BREAKFAST

2-egg omelette filled with vegetables, such as sautéed mixed onions, mushrooms and green peppers, and topped with 25g (1oz) grated reduced-fat Cheddar cheese

1 slice wholemeal toast with 1 teaspoon reduced-fat spread

175ml (6fl oz) calcium-fortified orange juice

Kcal: 490

AT-YOUR-DESK BREAKFAST

1 wholemeal mini bagel (7.5cm/3in) topped with 2 tablespoons peanut butter

1 medium banana

1 cup of black or green tea

Kcal: 449

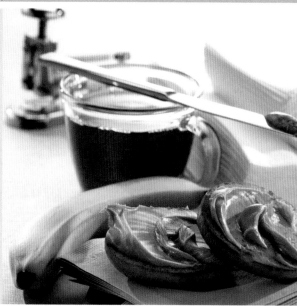

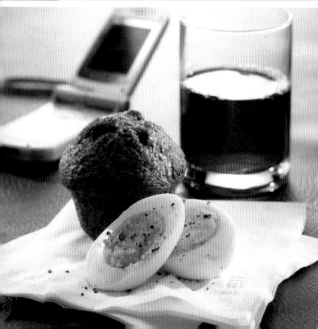

BRIEFCASE BREAKFAST

1 hard-boiled egg

1 low-fat Banana Bran Muffin (5cm/2in)
recipe on page 243

175ml (6fl oz) cranberry juice

Kcal: 300

Most of us have more leisure time at the weekend, so take advantage of it by whipping up a tasty, vegetable-filled omelette. Eggs provide plenty of protein and as much as half your daily quota of vitamin B_{12}, which may protect against diabetes-related neuropathy. Egg yolks also have modest amounts of zinc, which helps to protect cells in the pancreas that make insulin. No time to chop? Buy ready-cut vegetables.

TIPS

▶ For a lower-calorie omelette, use 1 egg and 2 egg whites. It will look and taste the same.

▶ Add or substitute vegetables in season, such as courgettes, broccoli or chopped spinach or tomatoes.

▶ Top with salsa and serve in a flour tortilla (forgo the toast) to make a breakfast wrap.

You dash off to work without breakfast. That's no problem – as long as you have emergency rations such as peanut butter and mini bagels or rice cakes in your desk drawer. Just grab a piece of fruit such as a banana on your way out the door. Peanut butter is an excellent protein source, although it's high in calories so stick to 2 tablespoons. Tea is rich in antioxidants that help to protect you from heart disease.

TIPS

▶ Beware of full-size bagels, which contain more carbohydrates and have twice the calories of 7.5cm (3in) bagels.

▶ If you're tired of bagels, substitute two rice cakes, which contain fewer calories. Rice cakes come in a variety of flavours, such as cinnamon and chocolate.

breakfast

Here's a meal you can pack and eat on your way. Just peel the egg before you leave the house and put it in a small polythene bag. If possible, bake your own muffins. Our recipe packs plenty of fibre and fruit with very little fat. If buying a muffin, choose one that is small and low in fat – some full-size muffins are gigantic calorie traps.

TIPS

▶ To enjoy eggs and protect your heart at the same time, buy eggs enhanced with omega-3 fatty acids – the same kind of fat found in oily fish such as salmon.

▶ As an alternative to fruit juice, enjoy some whole fruit, such as a handful of seedless red grapes.

▶ To cut calories further, choose light cranberry juice or other juices that are lower in sugar and calories.

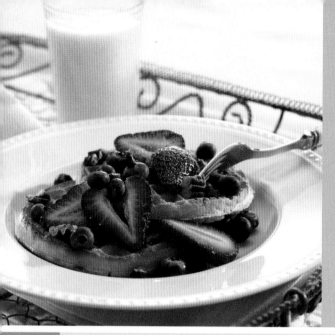

SPECIAL TREAT BREAKFAST

2 waffles topped with fresh fruit, such as blueberries and strawberries, and 1 tablespoon chopped pecan nuts

125ml (4fl oz) skimmed milk

Kcal: 350

BREAKFAST SANDWICH

1 fried egg between 2 English muffin halves, with sliced tomato and 25g (1oz) grated reduced-fat Cheddar cheese

175ml (6fl oz) orange juice

Kcal: 385

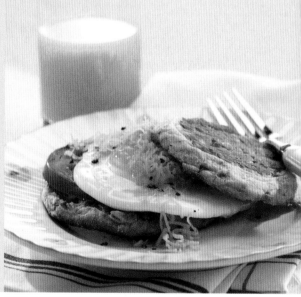

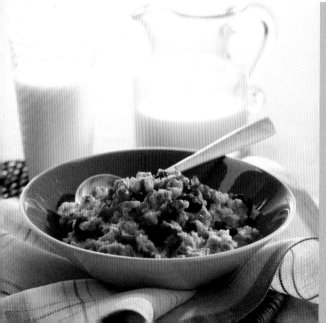

QUICK AND EASY WINTER WARMER

1 medium bowl of porridge, made with milk and water, topped with ½ teaspoon ground cinnamon, 2 tablespoons raisins and 1 tablespoon chopped walnuts

225ml (8fl oz) skimmed milk

Kcal: 400

Here's a sweet way to start the day. You may be surprised to see waffles, but in fact they can easily fit into the plan. Topping the waffles with fresh fruit instead of syrup and whipped cream avoids empty calories, and nuts add protein as well as heart-healthy monounsaturated fat.

TIPS

▶ Skip the milk and, for about the same number of calories, top the waffles and fruit with fat-free sugar-free yogurt.

▶ Make whole-grain or wholemeal waffles for a fibre bonus.

▶ Vary the types of fruit and nuts you put on top to keep breakfast interesting. Blueberries, strawberries, raspberries and other berries are loaded with antioxidants to fight off disease, so they offer a nutritional bonus.

This is just like a take-away breakfast, but with fewer calories and a serving of vegetables (the tomato). Choose wholemeal English muffins for extra fibre. If you haven't tasted reduced-fat cheese, give it a try. It's great for a breakfast dish like this.

TIPS

▶ Instead of frying the egg in butter or oil, use a non-stick frying pan with a little cooking spray.

▶ For an egg sandwich 'florentine' style, add some steamed spinach.

breakfast

You know porridge is good for you: it's loaded with fibre and removes bad cholesterol. But the biggest surprise benefit of this breakfast is that the cinnamon you add for flavour may naturally – and significantly – lower blood sugar in people with Type 2 diabetes. Cinnamon also gives the impression of sweetness without adding calories.

TIPS

▶ Cooking the porridge with some of the milk mixed with water will make the porridge taste creamier.

▶ Use jumbo porridge oats rather than regular for slightly more fibre and a heartier texture.

▶ Substitute slices of fresh banana or strawberries for the dried fruit.

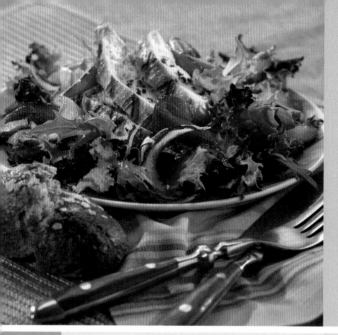

SAVOURY SALAD

2 to 3 handfuls of salad greens topped with 85g (3oz) chargrilled chicken and chargrilled vegetables such as red onions, portobello or chestnut mushrooms and red and green peppers

1 small wholegrain roll

Kcals: 350

lunch

CHAMPIONSHIP CHILLI

1 serving of Hearty Turkey Chilli
recipe on page 239

2 or 3 savoury wholemeal crackers

Kcal: 109

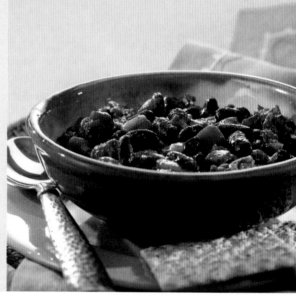

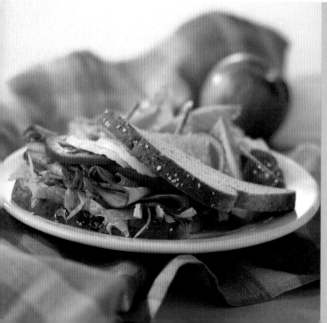

LUNCHBOX SPECIAL

55g (2oz) sliced turkey breast and 1 slice half-fat mozzarella cheese or reduced-fat Cheddar cheese on 2 slices whole-grain bread

Mixed salad with 1 tablespoon low-fat dressing

1 medium apple

Kcal: 370

This salad has it all: lean chicken breast for protein and plenty of antioxidant-rich vegetables. By chargrilling the vegetables, or cooking them under the grill, you bring out their rich flavour and natural sweetness. You can top the salad with 1 tablespoon of low-fat dressing if you like, although it has plenty of flavour on its own.

TIPS

▶ Instead of a roll, use a wholemeal flour tortilla and roll up the salad ingredients to make a tasty wrap.

▶ Other vegetables that are also great chargrilled are aubergine, courgettes and asparagus.

▶ No time to chargrill the veg? Then just open a jar of roasted peppers and one of artichoke hearts. Drain well and pat dry with kitchen paper before using.

High in fibre and low in fat, beans and other pulses are the perfect food for people with diabetes. And this chilli wins a top award for nutrition as it's made with minced turkey and plenty of vegetables. There's more than enough fibre and protein here to fill you up until dinner (with a small snack in between, of course!).

TIPS

▶ Substitute any type of beans you like for the kidney beans, such as black, pinto or cannellini beans.

▶ Soya mince will provide all the protein of minced turkey and the texture of minced meat. Why not try this meatless alternative for a change of pace, to cut saturated fat.

lunch

Add spice to a traditional packed lunch by filling your sandwich with extra-flavourful peppered turkey. With reduced-fat cheese and some mustard, you will have a sandwich with plenty of protein but almost no fat. The side salad and apple fill out the fruit and veg section of your balanced 'plate'.

TIPS

▶ For a hot version, grill the sandwich until the cheese melts.

▶ Replace the turkey with other sliced lean meat that has 3g of fat or less per serving.

▶ Instead of salad, pack some crudités such as peppers, celery and carrots.

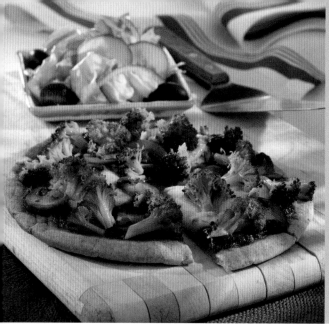

PITTA PIZZA

1 wholemeal pitta bread topped
   with blanched broccoli florets,
   55g (2oz) half-fat mozzarella and
   2 tablespoons tomato sauce, then
   baked briefly

Mixed salad with 1 tablespoon
   low-fat dressing

Kcal: 366

A TASTE OF FRANCE

1 serving of Tuna Salad Provençale
   recipe on page 225

Kcal: 223

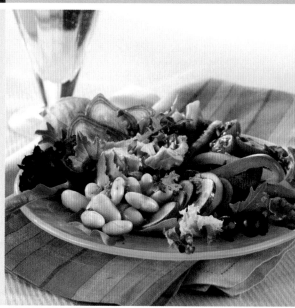

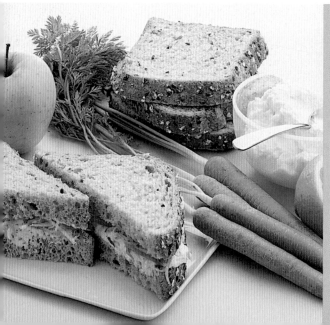

RICOTTA CRUNCH

2 heaped tablespoons ricotta cheese
   blended with 2 tablespoons each
   grated apple and carrot, plus lemon
   or orange juice to taste, and spread
   between 2 slices of oatmeal or
   multigrain bread

Kcal: 270

Who says you can't have pizza? It's true that regular fat-laden pizza is off-limits, but it's ever so simple to make a healthy pizza at home. Topped with lots of vegetables, this is a perfect lunch when you're trying to control calories and blood sugar. If you opt for a ready-made pizza, choose one with a thin crust and a vegetable topping, and blot up excess oil with kitchen paper.

TIPS

▸ For a Tex-Mex pizza, spread a flour tortilla with red kidney beans, salsa and reduced-fat cheese. Microwave for 90 seconds, then top with shredded lettuce, chopped spring onions and a little more salsa or taco sauce.

▸ If you're heating up a frozen pizza that is light on vegetables, dress it up with sliced peppers, shredded spinach and chopped olives.

Full of fibre, this salad shows how a simple can of tuna can be transformed with the help of an all-star medley of vegetables and a can of cannellini beans. Canned tuna is rich in vitamin B_{12}, which helps protect people with diabetes from nerve damage.

TIPS

▸ Buy tuna canned in water, not oil. It has far fewer calories.

▸ For a special treat, use grilled fresh tuna instead of canned.

lunch

This sandwich offers a tangy taste with a fraction of the calories and fat usually found in a cheese sandwich. With creamy ricotta, there's no need for butter or spread, nor for mayonnaise or other high-fat condiments. And adding some fruit and veg to the sandwich filling provides a vitamin boost as well as a delightful crunch.

TIPS

▸ If you are going to pack the sandwich in the morning, put some lettuce leaves between the filling and bread to prevent sogginess.

▸ For an even lower-fat sandwich, use 8%-fat fromage frais instead of ricotta.

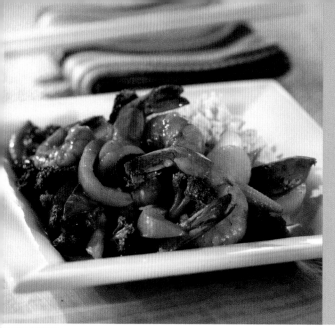

SUCCULENT STIR-FRY

1 serving of Prawn and Vegetable
Stir-Fry
recipe on page 222

50g (2oz) brown rice

Kcal: 431

dinner

MEAT-LOVER'S MEAL

140g (5oz) grilled lean rump steak

55g (2oz) sautéed button mushrooms

1 medium jacket-baked potato
topped with 2 tablespoons low-fat
cottage cheese or 0%-fat plain
Greek yogurt

1 serving of Courgette and
Tomato Gratin
recipe on page 230

Kcal: 588

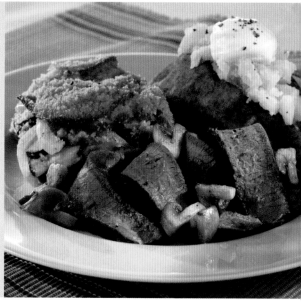

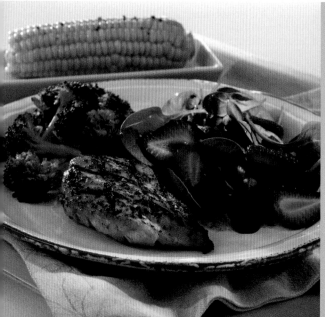

CAJUN SPICE

115g (4oz) grilled chicken breast fillet
rubbed with Cajun seasoning

Steamed broccoli

Green salad with sliced fresh
strawberries

1 corn-on-the-cob

Kcal: 300

Once maligned, prawns are actually a wonderful food – a good source of protein and very low in fat. And making stir-fries is a great way to get dinner on the table fast, especially if you buy pre-cut vegetables. For very busy nights, keep a ready-made prawn-and-vegetable meal on hand in the freezer and add extra frozen vegetables straight to the wok.

TIPS

▶ When choosing frozen ready meals, look for those that contain 300kcal or less and no more than 10g of fat and 800mg of sodium. Meals designed for slimmers usually fit the bill.

▶ For a bit more kick, add ½ teaspoon crushed dried chillies and 2 chopped spring onions.

▶ If you're watching your salt intake, always choose reduced-sodium soy sauce.

This meal is higher in calories than other dinner menus, but if you're a meat-and-potatoes kind of person, there's no reason you can't have them occasionally, as long as you keep calories under control at other times. The key here is choosing a lean cut of meat, limiting your portion to about 140g (5oz) and keeping your potato topping light.

TIPS

▶ Lower-fat cuts of beef include fillet, sirloin and rump (joints and steaks), as well as topside and thick flank or top rump.

▶ Steer clear of ribs and brisket.

▶ Trimmed venison, veal and lamb are generally lean.

dinner

When the weather is fine, cook the chicken on a barbecue. The corn can be cooked over the coals too – leave it in its green husk, and soak in water for 2 hours beforehand. Barbecue for 10–15 minutes, turning regularly. With some green veg and a salad brightened with fresh strawberries, you've got a colourful, casual meal that's perfect for outdoor eating.

TIPS

▶ Instead of corn-on-the-cob, have a small jacket potato. It will cook on the barbecue (wrapped in foil) in about the same time as the chicken.

▶ Splash the salad with balsamic vinegar. It goes well with strawberries and adds very few calories.

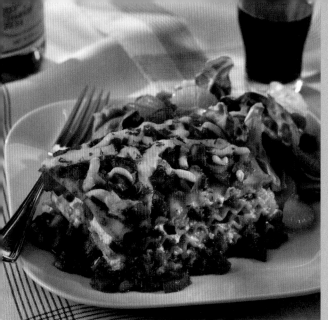

IT HAS TO BE PASTA

10cm (4in) square piece of
    vegetable lasagne

Mixed salad with orange segments
    and 1 tablespoon low-fat dressing

Kcal: 600

dinner

OMEGA GLORY

175g (6oz) baked or grilled
    salmon fillet

Greens sautéed in 1 teaspoon extra
    virgin olive oil

Steamed carrots

1 serving of Lemon Barley with
    Sultanas
    recipe on page 237

Kcal: 540

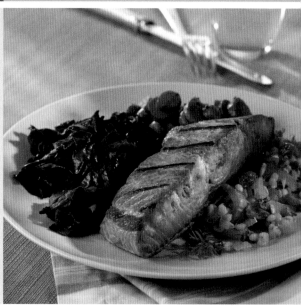

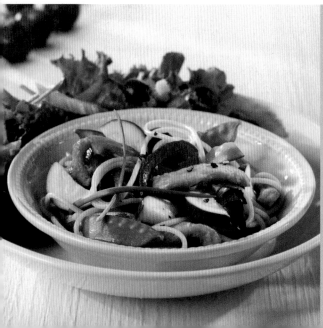

PERFECT PRIMAVERA

Fresh or frozen stir-fry vegetables
    sautéed in 1 tablespoon extra virgin
    olive oil with garlic, then tossed
    with 85g (3oz) cooked sliced
    chicken fillet and 4oz (115g)
    spaghetti; finished with 1 teaspoon
    freshly grated Parmesan cheese

Mixed salad with 1 tablespoon
    low-fat dressing

Kcal: 360

If you've been avoiding lasagne because of its fat content, put the ingredients for a meatless version on your shopping list: vegetables add colour and bulk without the fat of meat. Toss orange segments into your salad for a burst of colour and sweetness.

TIPS

▶ Thawed frozen spinach and roasted peppers, courgettes and aubergine make excellent fillings for lasagne.

▶ To satisfy meat lovers, add soya mince or Quorn, which mimic the texture and appearance of meat without the fat.

▶ Lasagne freezes well, so make double. Bake the second lasagne in a disposable aluminium baking tin, then seal with foil before freezing.

The omega-3 fatty acids in oily fish are so good for you that recommendations are to eat fish at least two times a week. Sautéed Swiss chard, kale and spring greens provide a whopping dose of magnesium (low levels may be linked with diabetes), the antioxidant beta-carotene and over 25 per cent of the RDA of vitamin C. And barley is a rich source of cholesterol-lowering soluble fibre.

TIPS

▶ For a change of pace, try mackerel, which is another good source of omega-3s.

▶ Not a fan of leafy greens? Substitute green beans sprinkled with almonds.

dinner

You can make this meal using fresh vegetables, but it's fine to substitute frozen stir-fry vegetables if you don't have much time. Just fry the vegetables quickly in a small amount of oil with a little garlic, toss in a bit of leftover grilled chicken and sprinkle with Parmesan cheese.

TIPS

▶ For the best flavour, buy a block of Parmesan cheese and grate it as you need it.

▶ Substitute chopped fresh asparagus or spinach for the mixed stir-fry vegetables.

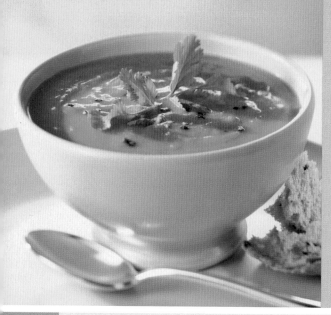

KEEP OUT THE CHILL

1 serving of Spiced Pumpkin and
    Bacon Soup
    recipe on page 240

1 crusty bread roll

Mixed salad with walnuts and raisins
    and 1 tablespoon low-fat dressing

Kcal: 380

dinner

PORK CHOPS TONIGHT

150g (5½oz) grilled or baked pork
    loin chop

Steamed green beans with flaked
    almonds

1 small potato, sliced and roasted
    with 1 teaspoon olive oil

Kcal: 403

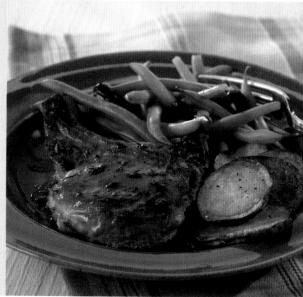

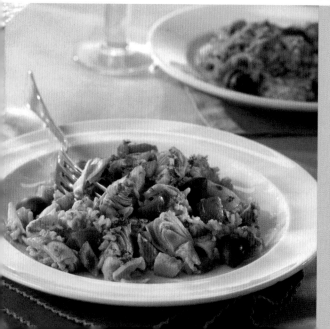

EASY PILAF

1 serving of Crab and Artichoke Rice
    recipe on page 223

Steamed asparagus spears

Kcal: 255

When the weather outside is dreadful, nothing's better than a hearty main-dish soup. It's an ideal way to get the robust flavour of meat – here lean smoked back bacon – without eating a lot of it. This thick, savoury soup, enlivened with aromatic cumin, is really satisfying, and the bread roll and salad make up a well-balanced and nutritious meal.

TIPS

▶ Instead of pumpkin, try using a squash such as butternut or kabocha. Butternut squash has a sweeter taste and smoother texture than pumpkin; kabocha squash has a drier texture and paler flesh.

▶ Rashers of back bacon, trimmed of fat, are much leaner than streaky bacon and give a fantastic flavour to this soup.

Pork loin is one of the leanest cuts of meat you can buy – if you trim off any visible fat, it's almost as lean as chicken breast. Pork contains zinc, which helps protect the insulin-making cells in the pancreas. A baked dessert apple sprinkled with cinnamon – which may help control blood sugar – would be the perfect ending to this meal.

TIPS

▶ To ensure juicy pork, choose a thick chop rather than a thin one.

▶ Sprinkle the chop with fresh or dried thyme for extra flavour.

▶ If you like, substitute veal loin chops, which are also very lean.

▶ For more nutrients and a slower rise in blood sugar, have a small, jacket-baked sweet potato instead. Be sure to eat the skin, which contains most of the fibre and nutrients.

dinner

This sophisticated dish isn't cooked as much as assembled, which makes it super fast and easy. All of the protein, vegetables and carbohydrates you need are here in one dish. And the health benefits are considerable: crab is low in fat and loaded with zinc, an important mineral for people with diabetes. Make it with brown rice instead of white to keep your blood sugar steadier.

TIPS

▶ Consider using cooked peeled prawns or cubed cooked chicken breast instead of crabmeat.

▶ Add red and yellow peppers for an appealing splash of colour and extra nutrients, such as vitamins C and A.

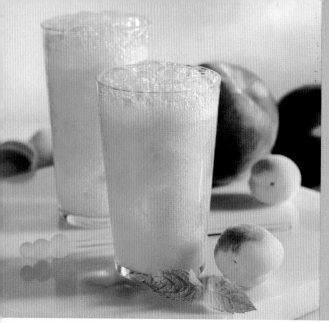

FRAGRANT FIZZ

Fresh fruit fizz (whiz the flesh from ¼ ripe mango, ¼ ripe peach and ½ large ripe apricot with 125ml/ 4fl oz low-calorie ginger ale until smooth and frothy)

Kcal: 47

This refreshing fruit drink provides a feast of vitamins. It's also great made with low-calorie bitter lemon instead of ginger ale.

desserts

ICE CREAM SUNDAE

3–4 small scoops of reduced-fat vanilla ice cream or frozen yogurt

1 serving of Hot Plum Sauce
recipe on page 244

Kcal: 190

At any time of year, you're sure to have ice cream on your mind. By choosing low-fat ice cream or frozen yogurt and topping with a fresh fruit sauce, you can cut the calories enough to indulge.

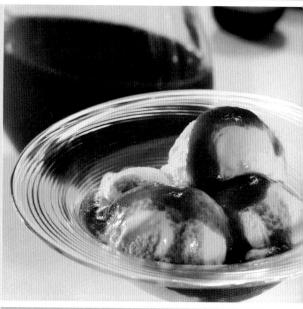

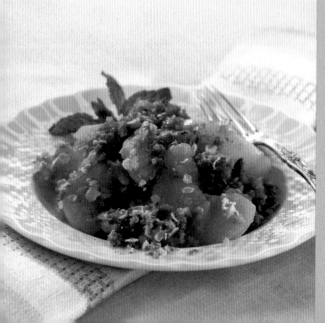

PEACHY KEEN

1 serving of Peach Crisp
recipe on page 246

Kcal: 140

Sweet, spicy and crunchy – this dessert has it all (and healthy fruit too). Using reduced-fat spread instead of butter helps to keep the calories in check, and oats provide fibre to keep blood sugar from rising too quickly.

MELON MELODY

3 slices each of honeydew melon,
   Charentais melon and mango

Kcal: 35

As with a simple song, the biggest
pleasure sometimes comes from the
clear flavours of just a few elements.
With melons carrying the tune and
mango providing a lively harmony,
this dessert is pared to the basics yet
is still elegant and delightful.

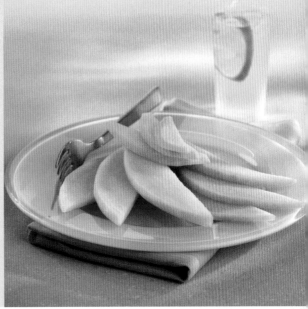

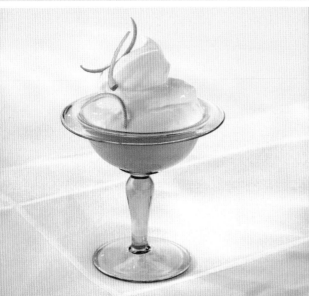

CITRUS CREAM

1 serving of Lemon-Lime
   Yogurt Mousse
   recipe on page 244

Kcal: 138

This simple mousse – deliciously
sweet yet tangy – is made with sugar-
free citrus jelly and yogurt and
topped with airy whipped cream. It's
a real treat.

desserts

CHOCS AWAY

1 serving of Chocolate-Banana
   Pudding Parfait
   recipe on page 244

Kcal: 146

If you serve this to friends, you'll
have to reassure them that you are
still eating healthily. Made with sugar-
free chocolate pudding mix and
whipped cream, it tastes infinitely
more sinful than it is.

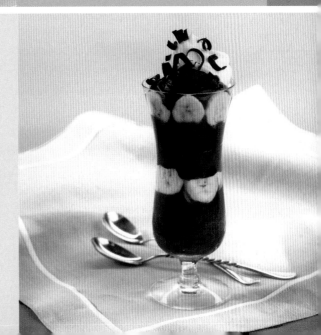

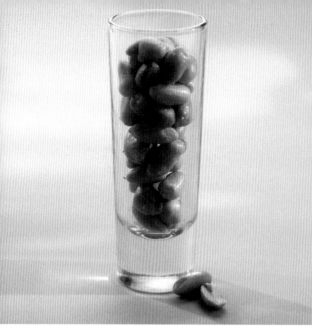

LET'S GO NUTS

25g (1oz) peanuts

Kcal: 141

The shopper in you will appreciate the dense, filling goodness you can get from a relatively small serving of peanuts. Full of protein and 'good' fats, nuts actually appear to help people lose weight. Feel free to substitute a palmful of almonds or a tablespoon of peanut butter.

TORTILLAS AND SALSA

1 crisp-baked corn tortilla with a fruity salsa dip

Kcal: 150

Cut corn tortillas into wedges and bake at 160°C (325°F, gas mark 3) for 15 minutes or until crisp. Cool, then serve with a vitamin-rich salsa of diced mangoes and ripe tomatoes with green chilli, garlic, lime juice and fresh coriander to taste.

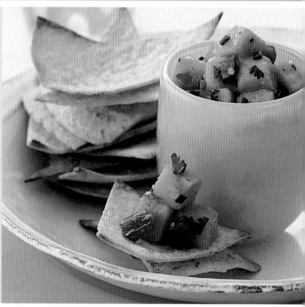

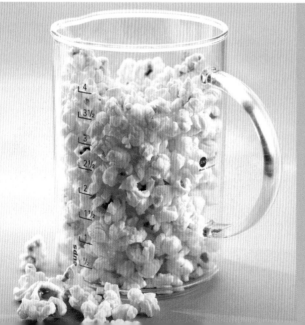

CINEMATIC LICENSE

3 handfuls of air-popped popcorn

Kcal: 100

Who says popcorn is only for the cinema? Take popcorn out of the multiplex and have it as a light snack any time. It's low in calories (as long as you don't add butter or a syrup) and high in fibre.

DARE TO BE GRAPE

20 seedless red grapes

Kcal: 36

Grapes are full of water, which makes them automatically low in calories. Twenty grapes registers in your brain as lots of separate items – popping them into your mouth one by one makes you feel that you're getting more than you really are.

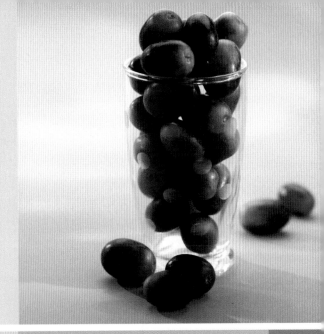

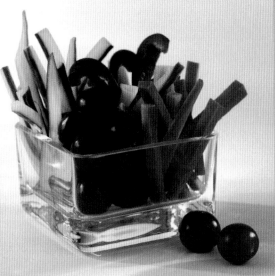

VEG VARIETY

Mixed vegetable crudités, such as 5 cherry tomatoes, ½ carrot and ¼ red pepper

Kcal: 40

Think of vegetables as sociable foods: they hate to be alone. Even when you snack, you'll have a livelier time if you mix veg together and let their tastes and textures mingle. Soft and crunchy, juicy and dense, mixed crudités are colourful too.

snacks

A CHERRY JUBILEE

85g (3oz) cherries

Kcal: 40

Fresh sweet cherries have a very low GI and they provide good amounts of vitamin C. They also contain phytochemicals called anthocyanins, which are believed to help keep the heart healthy.

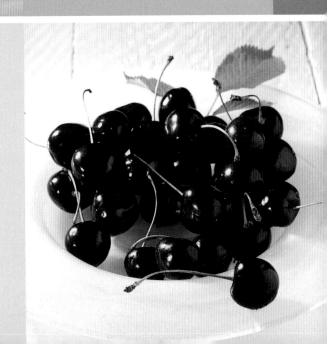

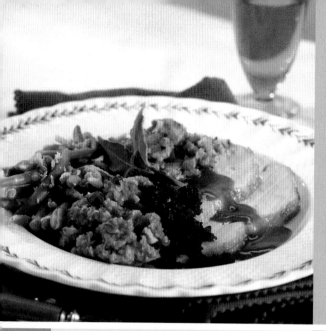

CHRISTMAS DINNER

150g (5½oz) roast turkey breast with
   2 tablespoons gravy and
   2 tablespoons cranberry relish

1 serving of Sage and Onion Stuffing
   recipe on page 236

1 serving of Praline-Sweet
   Potato Casserole
   recipe on page 236

1 serving of Easy Green Bean Casserole
   recipe on page 230

Kcal: 595

special menus

SUNDAY LUNCH

150g (5½oz) lean baked ham

1 serving of Scalloped Potatoes
   recipe on page 234

1 serving of Rosemary Peas
   and Onions
   recipe on page 231

1 serving of Waldorf Salad
   recipe on page 233

Kcal: 485

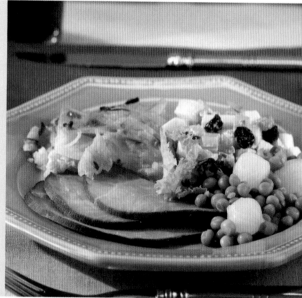

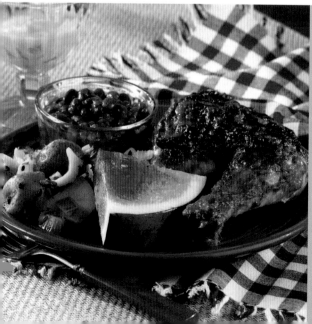

SUMMER BARBECUE

225g (8oz) Barbecued Chicken
   recipe on page 219

1 serving of German-style
   Potato Salad
   recipe on page 234

'Barbecued' baked beans

1 slice watermelon 7.5cm (3in) thick

1 serving of Tropical Fruit Pudding
   recipe on page 246

Kcal: 617

After Christmas dinner you often feel uncomfortably full, but it's easy to enjoy the feast without overdoing it. Turkey is traditionally the centrepiece, which is fine because it's low in fat – as long as you stick to white meat and keep the portion size to a reasonable 175g (6oz). To accompany the turkey, try the dishes in this menu – all were specially designed to be lower in fat and calories.

TIPS

▶ Don't be tempted by crisps or other salty snacks beforehand. Instead, munch a healthy snack such as celery sticks. (You'll probably have celery left over from making the stuffing.)

▶ Avoid Christmas pudding; it's a virtual calorie bomb. Choose Apple Pie (page 125) or Pear and Redcurrant Lattice (page 247) instead.

The savoury smell of lean baked ham filling the air is just part of what makes this meat perfect for Sunday lunch. Both lean and succulent, ham has an abundance of flavour but can be sliced thin to keep taste satisfaction high and calories low. The accompanying dishes are perfect complements to the ham, making a colourful and satisfying meal.

TIPS

▶ If you're going to drink wine, enjoy it with lunch rather than beforehand, and have a glass of water alongside. That way, the alcohol won't weaken your resolve not to overeat, plus you'll drink fewer empty calories.

▶ Can't resist the mixed nuts? Fill the bowl with nuts in their shells and use a traditional nutcracker. The effort will slow you down and make you more mindful of how much you're eating.

special menus

As soon as the sun shines, get out the barbecue and wow your friends and family with this barbecued chicken. The aromas will be irresistible. Serve with special potato salad, sweet melon and extra-savoury baked beans (mix canned beans with the sauce reserved from the chicken and heat in a saucepan next to the chicken on the barbecue). Finish with an easy creamy pudding.

TIPS

▶ Removing the skin from chicken cuts calories significantly.

▶ To cut barbecuing time (and ensure that the chicken is thoroughly cooked), partly cook the breasts first in the microwave, on high for 3–4 minutes.

STEP 4

Master your disaster foods

A key aspect of the 10 Per Cent Plan is that you never have to do without foods you love. (Otherwise, frankly, the chances that you'd stick with the plan would be slim.) If you are like most people, though, many of the dishes on your list of favourites are dietary disasters loaded with fat and calories. An insurmountable problem? Hardly.

On the following pages, you'll find recipes for more than a dozen classic favourites, from burgers and chips to pizza and cheesecake, that have been modified to substantially reduce fat and calories while preserving the flavours you love.

It's time to stop thinking of good-tasting food as a stumbling block. If you love macaroni cheese or chicken wings, you don't have to deprive yourself. These lower-calorie versions let you indulge – in moderation, of course – without the guilt.

How can you take a meal such as a burger and chips and make it better for you? The most obvious answer is to cut some of the dietary fat which, weight for weight, contains more than twice as many calories as carbohydrate or protein. (It will also help to keep portions small and round out your meal with plenty of vegetables.)

In fact, fat gets more credit for taste than it deserves. In many cases, it's texture you want (creamy, meaty, crunchy), not the fat itself. In other cases, fat is simply an ingredient that happens to come with some foods, such as dairy products and certain cuts of meat, but not others.

We pared these worst-offender recipes of much of their fat content and included a few other key calorie-saving changes as well. The good thing is, you still get great taste. And you can easily give the same treatment to other favourite foods. Simply follow these guidelines.

- Substitute leaner meats for fattier ones, such as white-meat poultry for dark, lean minced turkey for minced beef, or pork tenderloins for ribs.

- Bake or grill instead of frying in oil, which saturates the food you are cooking, especially if the food is breaded.

- Remove skin from poultry and trim visible fat from meat. Why worry about hidden fat when the fat you can see – and remove – does most of the harm?

- Buy low-fat or sugar-free products. If you haven't recently tried low-fat or fat-free foods (especially cheese), try them again: they have improved. If one brand doesn't taste good to you, try another. And you will always save calories by using naturally lower-fat cheeses such as mozzarella or cottage cheese instead of higher-fat ones such as Cheddar.

- Mix higher-fat meats, cheeses and other foods with lower-fat versions if you don't want to make complete substitutions.

Cutting a few calories at every meal will add up to real calorie savings. Once you have cut 3,500kcal, you will have lost 500g (1lb) of fat. Now, to find specific solutions for some of your favourite foods, turn to the recipes on the next few pages.

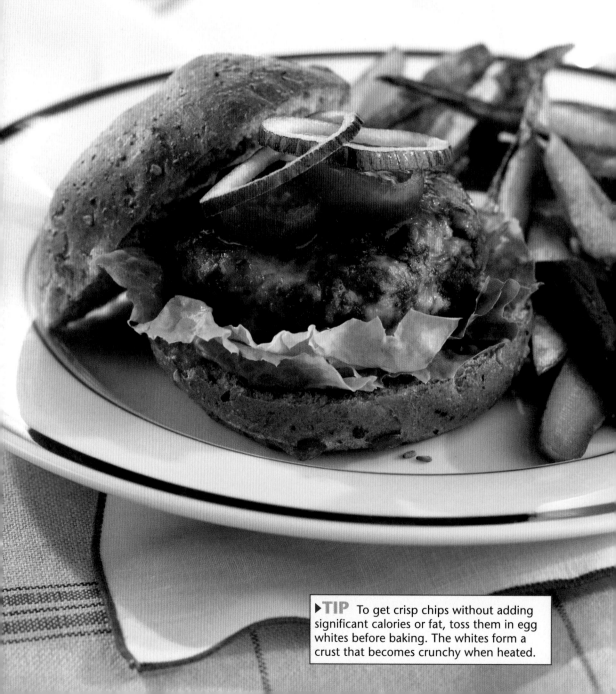

▶TIP Whole-grain burger buns provide fibre as do wholemeal buns. If you prefer to use white burger buns, choose those that are labelled 'lite', 'light', or 'diet'. These will have fewer calories than regular white burger buns.

▶TIP To get crisp chips without adding significant calories or fat, toss them in egg whites before baking. The whites form a crust that becomes crunchy when heated.

Hamburgers

SERVES 6

The classic hamburger is usually avoided in a healthy eating plan, because a third of the typical burger's calories comes from saturated fat. But you can make this favourite meal dramatically healthier by choosing leaner beef and mixing it with minced turkey, and bulking up the meat with mushrooms and high-fibre oats.

225g (8oz) very lean minced beef

225g (8oz) minced turkey

40g (1½oz) mushrooms, finely chopped

20g (¾oz) porridge oats or fresh breadcrumbs

2 tablespoons finely chopped onion

6 wholegrain burger buns

Lettuce, tomato slices and red onion rings

1. Combine the beef, turkey, mushrooms, oats or crumbs and onion in a large bowl. Form into 6 burgers.

2. Grill or barbecue the burgers until cooked through. Serve on the buns with lettuce, tomato and red onion.

DISASTER FOOD	MASTER FOOD
450g (1lb) regular minced beef	225g (8oz) each very lean minced beef and minced turkey with oats and chopped mushrooms
Regular burger bun	Wholegrain burger bun
Kcal per serving: 315	Kcal per serving: 251
Fat per serving: 14g	Fat per serving: 6g

Oven chips

SERVES 2

What burger is complete without chips? The trouble is that soft-fleshed potatoes are grease sponges, and deep-frying more than triples calories. The solution is to make chips satisfyingly crisp by baking them in a high heat.

1 medium potato, about 175g (6oz)

Salt (optional)

1. Pierce the potato, then microwave for about 4 minutes. Set aside until cool enough to handle.

2. Preheat the oven to 240°C (475°F, gas mark 9) or its highest setting. Spray a baking tray with cooking spray.

3. Cut the potato into strips, leaving on the skin, and arrange in a single layer on the baking tray. Lightly spray the tops with cooking spray and sprinkle with salt, if using.

4. Bake for about 10 minutes, turning once, until the chips are brown and crisp.

DISASTER FOOD	MASTER FOOD
Deep-fried chips	Oven-baked chips
Cooked in oil	Coated with cooking spray
Kcal per serving: 263	Kcal per serving: 93
Fat per serving: 22g	Fat per serving: 3g

master your disaster foods

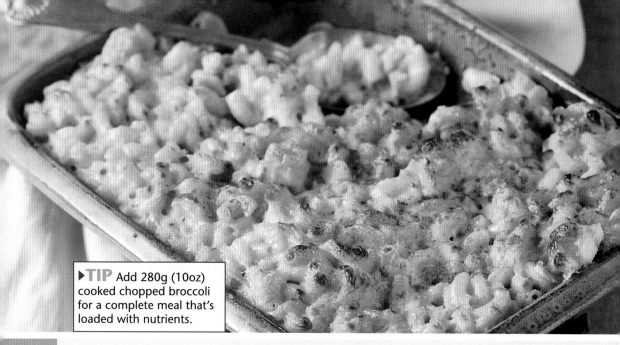

> ▶**TIP** Add 280g (10oz) cooked chopped broccoli for a complete meal that's loaded with nutrients.

Macaroni cheese

SERVES 6

You probably never thought that a creamy dish could be low in fat, but this version is. Calorie savings, though significant, aren't enormous, but you dramatically cut the saturated fat – the dangerous kind that makes blood sugar control more difficult and increases the risk of heart disease.

40g (1½oz) reduced-fat spread

4 tablespoons plain flour

¾ teaspoon mustard powder

2 cans (about 400g each) light evaporated milk

25g (1oz) Parmesan cheese, freshly grated

115g (4oz) reduced-fat mature Cheddar cheese, grated

½ teaspoon salt

¼ teaspoon freshly ground black pepper

675g (1½lb) cooked short-cut macaroni

Pinch of paprika

1. Preheat the oven to 180°C (350°F, gas mark 4). Lightly grease a large baking dish.

2. Melt the spread in a large, heavy saucepan over low heat. Add the flour and stir until blended.

3. Add the mustard. Gradually add the evaporated milk, stirring constantly with a wire whisk. Cook over a moderate heat, stirring, for 12 minutes or until slightly thickened and bubbling. Remove from the heat.

4. Add the Parmesan, Cheddar, salt and pepper, and stir until the cheese melts.

5. Stir in the macaroni, then pour into the baking dish. Sprinkle lightly with the paprika. Bake for about 30 minutes or until bubbling. Serve hot.

DISASTER FOOD	MASTER FOOD
40g (1½oz) butter	40g (1½oz) reduced-fat spread
450ml (16fl oz) whole milk	2 cans (400g each) light evaporated milk
225g (8oz) full-fat Cheddar	115g (4oz) reduced-fat Cheddar and 25g (1oz) Parmesan
Kcal per serving: 425	Kcal per serving: 380
Fat per serving: 22g	Fat per serving: 14g

Aubergine parmigiana

When aubergine is coated with crumbs and fried, its sponginess makes it soak up the fat. This baked version, however, is wonderfully cheesy and saucily seasoned, and has two-thirds fewer calories than traditional recipes.

2 aubergines, peeled and sliced 1cm (½in) thick

2 teaspoons finely chopped garlic

Salt and freshly ground black pepper

450ml (16fl oz) marinara or tomato-based pasta sauce

115g (4oz) half-fat mozzarella cheese, grated

55g (2oz) dried breadcrumbs

25g (1oz) Parmesan cheese, freshly grated

1 tablespoon chopped parsley

1. Preheat the grill to high and the oven to 190°C (375°F, gas mark 5). Spray a large, rectangular baking dish with cooking spray.

2. Sprinkle the aubergine with the garlic and salt and pepper to taste. Arrange the slices in a single layer on a baking tray and spray with olive oil–flavoured cooking spray. Grill for 5 minutes on each side or until soft and lightly browned.

3. Layer one-third of the aubergine slices, sauce and mozzarella in the baking dish, then repeat the layers two more times. Sprinkle the top with the crumbs and Parmesan. Bake for about 30 minutes or until bubbling. Sprinkle with the parsley before serving.

DISASTER FOOD	MASTER FOOD
Deep–fried	Grilled and baked
Vegetable or olive oil	Olive oil–flavoured cooking spray
1 whole egg	No egg
175g (6oz) full-fat mozzarella	115g (4oz) half-fat mozzarella plus 25g (1oz) Parmesan
Kcal per serving: 213	Kcal per serving: 111
Fat per serving: 15g	Fat per serving: 5g

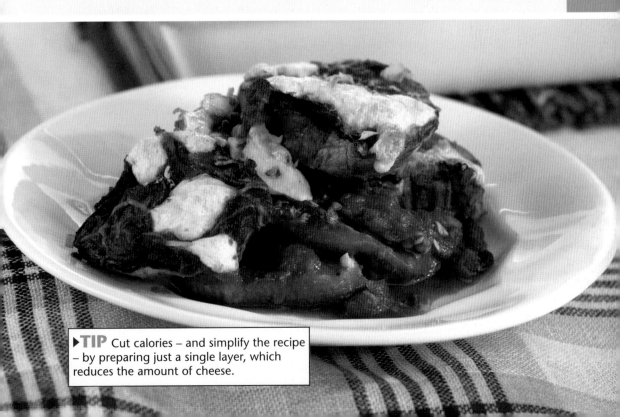

▶**TIP** Cut calories – and simplify the recipe – by preparing just a single layer, which reduces the amount of cheese.

'Fried' chicken

SERVES 6

Most of the problems with pan-fried chicken are only skin-deep. Pull off the skin, lighten the coating and bake rather than fry – you'll still have the crisp, savoury result you love.

6 skinless chicken breast fillets, about 675g (1½lb) in total

Salt and freshly ground black pepper

4 tablespoons skimmed milk

1 egg white, lightly beaten

50g (1¾oz) cornflakes, lightly crushed

1. Preheat the oven to 200°C (400°F, gas mark 6). Spray a baking tray with cooking spray.

2. Rinse the chicken and pat dry, then season with salt and pepper to taste.

3. Combine the milk and egg white in a shallow bowl. Place the cornflake crumbs on a plate. Dip each chicken piece in the egg and milk, then roll in the cornflake crumbs until evenly coated.

4. Arrange the chicken pieces in a single layer on the baking tray. Spray the tops with cooking spray, then bake for 20–30 minutes or until golden and crisp.

DISASTER FOOD	MASTER FOOD
Chicken pieces with skin, including dark meat	Chicken breast fillets without skin
Coated with beaten whole egg and breadcrumbs	Coated with egg white and cornflake crumbs
Fried in oil	Coated with cooking spray and baked
Kcal per serving: 342	Kcal per serving: 160
Fat per serving: 22g	Fat per serving: 2.5g

Mashed potatoes

SERVES 6

You can pare down the fat in this favourite dish with one smart substitution and a simple reduction. But don't undo your gains by smothering the potatoes with rich gravy! If you want more creaminess, add a modest amount of 0%-fat Greek yogurt instead.

900g (2lb) potatoes

175ml (6fl oz) skimmed milk, warmed

25g (1oz) butter

Salt and freshly ground black pepper to season

1. Peel the potatoes, place in a saucepan and add enough water to cover. Bring to the boil and cook for 15–20 minutes or until the potatoes are soft. Drain in a colander, then tip into a bowl.

2. Beat the potatoes with an electric mixer until smooth.

3. Add 125ml (4fl oz) of the milk and the butter, and season to taste with salt and pepper. Continue beating until the mash is fluffy, adding more milk if necessary to reach the desired consistency.

DISASTER FOOD	MASTER FOOD
40g (1½oz) or more butter	25g (1oz) butter
Whole milk or cream	Skimmed milk
Kcal per serving: 212	Kcal per serving: 153
Fat per serving: 10g	Fat per serving: 4g

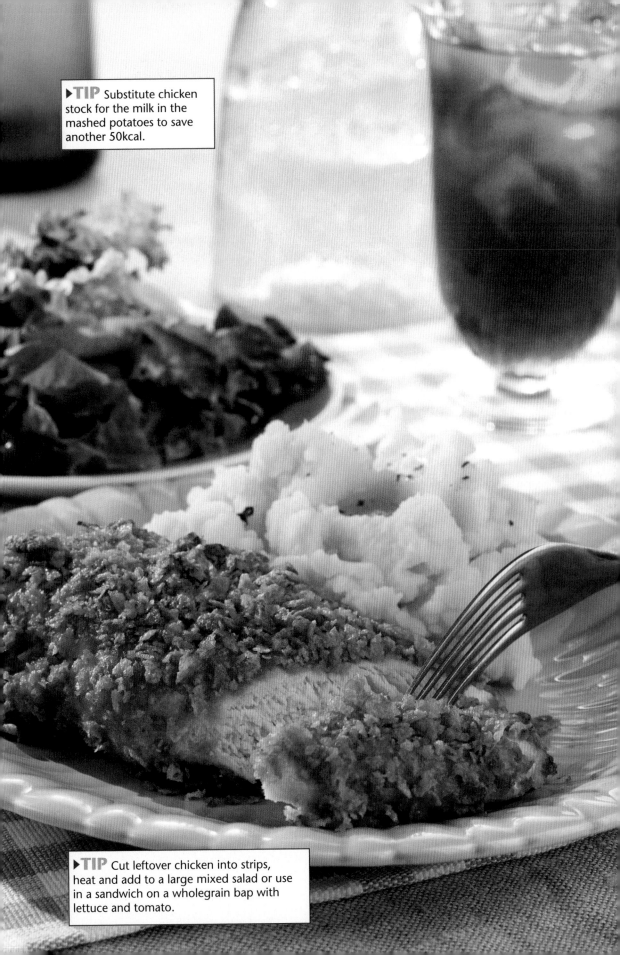

▶**TIP** Substitute chicken stock for the milk in the mashed potatoes to save another 50kcal.

▶**TIP** Cut leftover chicken into strips, heat and add to a large mixed salad or use in a sandwich on a wholegrain bap with lettuce and tomato.

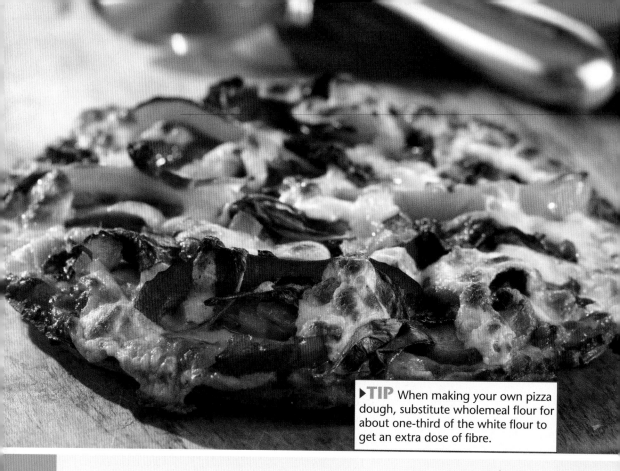

> ▶**TIP** When making your own pizza dough, substitute wholemeal flour for about one-third of the white flour to get an extra dose of fibre.

Vegetarian pizza

SERVES 4

A thin crust, lower-fat cheese and plenty of vegetables make this pizza a less guilty pleasure. Crumbled vegetarian sausages will give you all the savoury taste of meat sausage but almost none of the fat.

- 1 packet (about 280g) pizza base mix
- 225ml (8fl oz) tomato-based pizza or pasta sauce
- 4 vegetarian Quorn sausages, removed from casing if necessary
- 150g (5½oz) red peppers, cut into thin strips
- 40g (1½oz) mushrooms, thinly sliced
- 2 tablespoons chopped onion
- 85g (3oz) thawed frozen chopped spinach, well drained
- 85g (3oz) half-fat mozzarella cheese, grated

1. Preheat the oven to 230°C (450°F, gas mark 8). Spray a baking sheet with cooking spray.

2. Prepare the pizza dough according to the packet instructions. Press the dough into a thin 30cm (12in) round on the baking sheet. Spread the sauce evenly on the crust and crumble the sausages over the sauce. Top with the peppers, mushrooms, onion and spinach. Sprinkle with the cheese.

3. Bake for 12–17 minutes or until the crust is brown and the cheese is melted and golden.

DISASTER FOOD	MASTER FOOD
225g (8oz) or more full-fat mozzarella	85g (3oz) half-fat mozzarella
Pork sausage	Vegetarian sausage
Pepperoni	Peppers, mushrooms, onions, spinach
Kcal per serving*: 563	Kcal per serving*: 372
Fat per serving*: 25g	Fat per serving*: 7g
*2 slices	

Spicy chicken strips

This is inspired by a recipe for chicken wings coated with a zesty sauce, which was created in a New York pub 40 years ago. By substituting strips of lean, skinless chicken breast for high-fat wings, you'll keep the spicy flavour but lose most of the fat.

1 tablespoon vegetable oil

450g (1lb) skinless chicken breast fillets, cut into strips

2 tablespoons Tabasco sauce

1½ teaspoons cider vinegar

Salt and freshly ground black pepper

1. Heat the oil in a medium non-stick frying pan. Add the chicken and brown over moderate heat for about 5 minutes. Turn and cook for a further 3 minutes to brown the other side.

2. Sprinkle the Tabasco sauce and vinegar over the chicken and continue cooking for about 5 minutes. Increase the heat to high and cook for 2 minutes or until the chicken is coated and the sauce is completely reduced. Season with the salt and pepper to taste.

DISASTER FOOD	MASTER FOOD
Chicken wings	Skinless chicken breast fillet strips
25g (1oz) butter	1 tablespoon vegetable oil
Deep-fried and flavoured with sauce	Sautéed in vegetable oil with Tabasco sauce and vinegar
Kcal per serving: 360 for 115g (4oz) – about 12 large wings	Kcal per serving: 146 for 115g (4oz) – about 4 strips
Fat per serving: 20g	Fat per serving: 5g

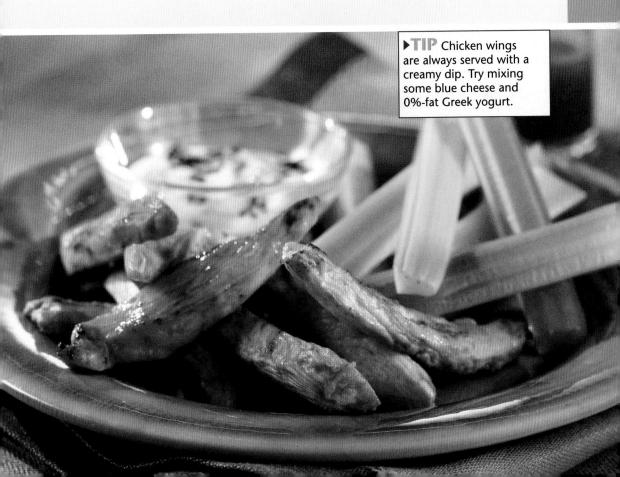

▶**TIP** Chicken wings are always served with a creamy dip. Try mixing some blue cheese and 0%-fat Greek yogurt.

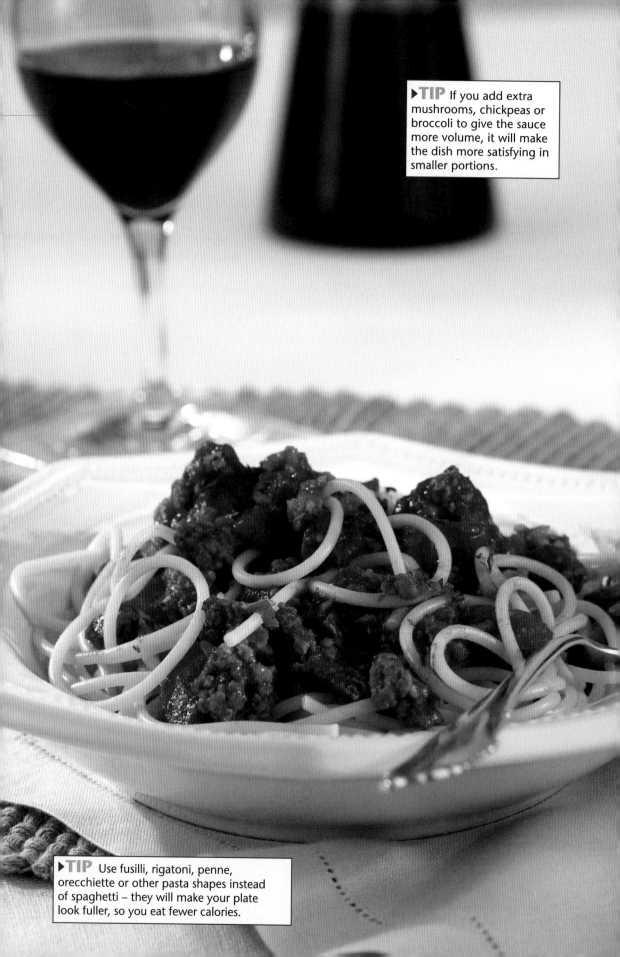

▶**TIP** If you add extra mushrooms, chickpeas or broccoli to give the sauce more volume, it will make the dish more satisfying in smaller portions.

▶**TIP** Use fusilli, rigatoni, penne, orecchiette or other pasta shapes instead of spaghetti – they will make your plate look fuller, so you eat fewer calories.

Spaghetti bolognese

Half the pleasure of a good bolognese sauce is its savoury taste and crumbly texture. Get the effect of a meaty mouthful by using less minced beef and adding soya mince. No one will notice the difference because soya mince looks and tastes like cooked minced beef in this rich tomato sauce. Or, as an alternative to soya, you could try 115g (4oz) lean minced turkey breast.

115g (4oz) very lean minced beef

200g (7oz) diced onion

35g (1¼oz) chopped green pepper

115g (4oz) soya mince or Quorn

1 teaspoon finely chopped garlic

85g (3oz) small button mushrooms, halved

115g (4oz) tomato sauce

2 cans (about 400g each) chopped tomatoes

1 tablespoon chopped parsley

½ teaspoon each dried thyme, basil and oregano

225g (8oz) spaghetti

1. Dry-fry the beef with the onion and green pepper in a medium non-stick frying pan for 5 minutes or until the beef is browned and crumbly, and the vegetables are softened.

2. Add the soya mince, garlic and mushrooms and cook for a further 3 minutes, stirring.

3. Add the tomato sauce, tomatoes, parsley and dried herbs. Simmer gently, stirring occasionally, for about 15 minutes.

4. Meanwhile, cook the spaghetti in boiling water until al dente. Drain and serve topped with the sauce.

DISASTER FOOD	MASTER FOOD
Regular minced beef	Lean minced beef and soya mince
225g (8oz) sausage	No sausage
Kcal per serving: 559	Kcal per serving: 335
Fat per serving: 25g	Fat per serving: 5g

master your disaster foods

'Fried' fish sandwich

High-protein fish is an excellent addition to your plate – but not when it's laden with oily batter and heavy helpings of mayonnaise. This finer fish dish solves those problems, providing only a fraction of the usual calories and fat without sacrificing crunch.

4 tablespoons skimmed milk

50g (1¾oz) cornflakes, coarsely crushed

2 teaspoons paprika

1 teaspoon lemon pepper

450g (1lb) white fish fillets, about 2.5cm (1in) thick, cut into fingers

4 seeded burger buns

1. Preheat the oven to 230°C (450°F, gas mark 8). Spray a baking tray with cooking spray.

2. Place the milk in a small bowl. Combine the cornflake crumbs, paprika and lemon pepper in a small bowl, then spread on a plate. Dip each fish finger in the milk, then coat with the seasoned crumbs. Place the fingers in a single layer on the baking tray.

3. Bake for about 10 minutes or until the fish flakes easily. Serve in the buns.

DISASTER FOOD	MASTER FOOD
Coated with egg batter	Coated with skimmed milk and cornflake crumbs
Deep-fried	Baked
Flavoured with mayonnaise or tartare sauce	Flavoured with lemon pepper and paprika
Kcal per serving: 574	Kcal per serving: 293
Fat per serving: 34g	Fat per serving: 3.5g

▶**TIP** Can't do without tartare sauce? Whip up a low-fat version using reduced-fat mayonnaise, finely diced dill-pickled gherkins and a little Dijon mustard.

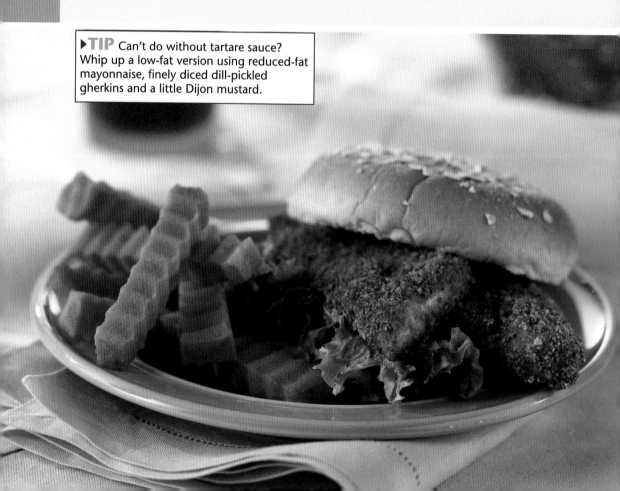

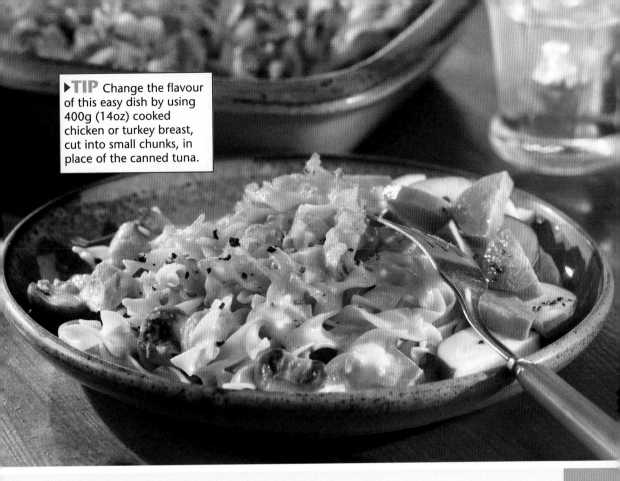

▶TIP Change the flavour of this easy dish by using 400g (14oz) cooked chicken or turkey breast, cut into small chunks, in place of the canned tuna.

Tuna and pasta bake

SERVES 4

This storecupboard dish could be loaded with fat, but that can easily be avoided with a few simple tweaks that won't significantly affect the creamy, savoury flavour.

225g (8oz) fusilli or wide egg noodles such as pappardelle

1 can (about 120g) button mushrooms, drained

1 can (about 300g) fat-free cream of mushroom soup

1 can (about 200g) tuna in water, drained

125ml (4fl oz) skimmed milk

115g (4oz) reduced-fat Cheddar cheese, grated

150g (5½oz) frozen peas

1. Preheat the oven to 180°C (350°F, gas mark 4).

2. Cook the pasta according to the packet instructions until al dente, then drain.

3. Combine the pasta, mushrooms, soup, tuna, milk, cheese and peas in a baking dish. Bake for about 30 minutes or until bubbling. Serve hot.

DISASTER FOOD	MASTER FOOD
1 can regular cream of mushroom soup	1 can fat-free cream of mushroom soup
2 cans tuna in oil	1 can tuna in water
2 eggs	No eggs
Whole milk	Skimmed milk
175g (6oz) grated full-fat Cheddar	115g (4oz) grated reduced-fat Cheddar
No vegetables	Frozen peas
Kcal per serving: 683	Kcal per serving: 437
Fat per serving: 34g	Fat per serving: 13g

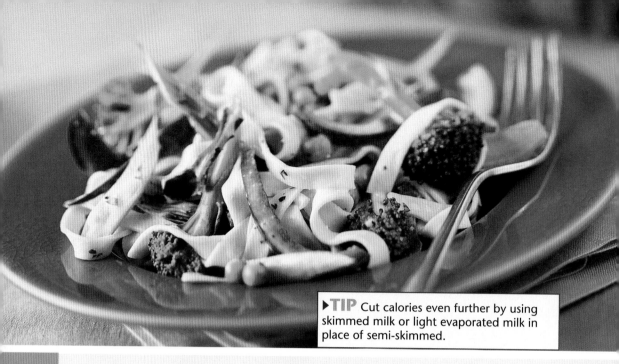

▸TIP Cut calories even further by using skimmed milk or light evaporated milk in place of semi-skimmed.

Fettuccine in cream sauce

SERVES 4

Lightening up the typical rich cream sauce and adding a medley of colourful vegetables makes this pasta dish healthy and appealing. The vegetables also bulk up the dish so you can eat more without increasing your calorie intake.

350g (12oz) fettuccine

200g (7oz) broccoli florets

225g (8oz) baby carrots, cut in half lengthways

150g (5½oz) shelled fresh or thawed frozen peas

1 large red pepper, deseeded and cut into thin strips

1 tablespoon reduced-fat spread

1 small garlic clove, finely chopped

2 tablespoons plain flour

½ teaspoon salt

350ml (12fl oz) semi-skimmed milk

125ml (4fl oz) reduced-fat single cream

50g (1¾oz) Parmesan cheese, freshly grated

1. Cook the fettuccine according to packet instructions until al dente. When ready, drain.

2. Meanwhile, bring a large saucepan of water to the boil. Cook the broccoli and carrots for 5 minutes. Add the peas and red pepper, and cook for a further 3 minutes. Drain and keep warm.

3. Melt the spread in a medium saucepan over moderate heat. Add the garlic and sauté for 1 minute or until golden. Whisk in the flour and salt, and cook for about 2 minutes or until bubbling. Gradually whisk in the milk and cream and bring to the boil. Reduce the heat and simmer, whisking constantly, for 1–2 minutes or until the sauce is thick.

4. Reduce the heat to low. Stir in the cheese until melted and smooth. Combine the fettuccine and vegetables with the sauce and serve immediately.

DISASTER FOOD	MASTER FOOD
No vegetables	Carrots, broccoli, peas, red pepper, garlic
Double cream	Reduced-fat single cream
Egg yolks	No egg
115g (4oz) Parmesan	50g (1¾oz) Parmesan
25g (1oz) butter	1 tablespoon reduced-fat spread
Kcal per serving: 783	Kcal per serving: 546
Fat per serving: 38g	Fat per serving: 14g

master your disaster foods

Burgundy beef stew

Using topside makes this dish much lower in fat than the traditional version using stewing steak. And because it's slow-cooked, the meat will be tender. Red wine gives flavour and colour as well as adding heart-protective antioxidants. A wealth of vegetables accented (not outnumbered) by cubes of beef keeps calories under control.

350g (12oz) beef topside, trimmed of all visible fat and cut into 1cm (½in) chunks

175g (6oz) thawed frozen button onions

3 carrots, thinly sliced

4 garlic cloves, slivered

1 tablespoon sugar

450g (1lb) chestnut mushrooms, quartered

2 tablespoons plain flour

125ml (4fl oz) dry red wine or chicken stock

175ml (6fl oz) water

¾ teaspoon dried thyme

¾ teaspoon salt

½ teaspoon freshly ground black pepper

1. Preheat the oven to 180°C (350°F, gas mark 4).

2. Spray a non-stick flameproof casserole with cooking spray. Add the beef and cook for about 5 minutes or until brown. Transfer to a plate with a slotted spoon.

3. Add the onions, carrots and garlic to the casserole. Sprinkle with the sugar and cook for about 7 minutes or until the onions are golden. Add the mushrooms and cook for a further 4 minutes or until tender.

4. Return the beef (and any accumulated juices) to the casserole. Sprinkle over the flour and cook, stirring, for about 3 minutes or until the flour has been absorbed.

5. Add the wine or stock and bring to the boil. Add the water, thyme, salt and pepper, and return to the boil. Cover and transfer to the oven. Cook for 1 hour or until the beef is tender. (The stew can be made ahead and refrigerated; reheat at 160°C/325°F, gas mark 3.)

DISASTER FOOD	MASTER FOOD
Stewing beef browned in oil	Topside browned with cooking spray
175g (6oz) beef per serving	85g (3oz) beef per serving
Potatoes	No potatoes and more vegetables
Kcal per serving: 551	Kcal per serving: 250
Fat per serving: 15g	Fat per serving: 7g

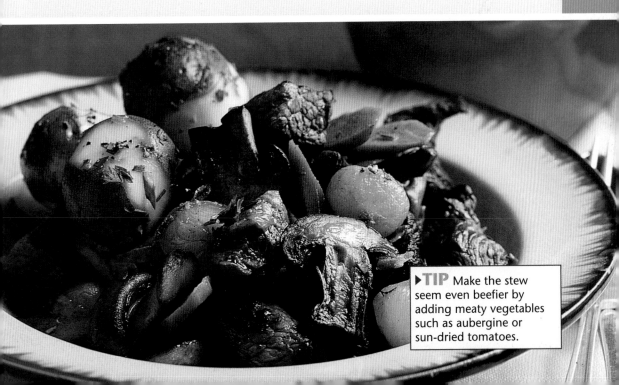

▶TIP Make the stew seem even beefier by adding meaty vegetables such as aubergine or sun-dried tomatoes.

master your disaster foods

Turkey enchiladas

Typically made with beef, this zesty recipe for corn tortillas filled and baked with a salsa and cheese topping cuts fat by substituting turkey and adding black beans. Fresh coriander and cumin enhance the Tex-Mex flavours.

600ml (1 pint) salsa

4 tablespoons chopped fresh coriander

1 teaspoon ground cumin

8 corn tortillas (15cm/6in)

225g (8oz) skinless cooked turkey breast, shredded

125g (4½ oz) canned black beans, rinsed and drained

1 small red onion, finely chopped

115g (4oz) reduced-fat Cheddar cheese, grated

1. Preheat the oven to 180°C (350°F, gas mark 4). Lightly spray a baking dish with cooking spray.

2. Combine the salsa, coriander and cumin in a shallow bowl that is at least 15cm (6in) in diameter.

3. Dip a tortilla in the salsa mixture, coating it completely. Place on a plate. Top with 2 tablespoons of the salsa mixture, then with one-eighth of the turkey, beans and onion. Sprinkle with 1 tablespoon of the cheese. Roll up and place seam-side down in the baking dish. Repeat with the remaining tortillas.

4. Spoon the remaining salsa mixture over the enchiladas and sprinkle with the remaining cheese. Bake for about 15 minutes or until bubbling. Serve hot.

DISASTER FOOD	MASTER FOOD
Beef chuck	Shredded turkey breast
Full-fat Cheddar	Reduced-fat Cheddar
No beans	Black beans
Kcal per serving: 661	Kcal per serving: 609
Fat per serving: 19g	Fat per serving: 10g

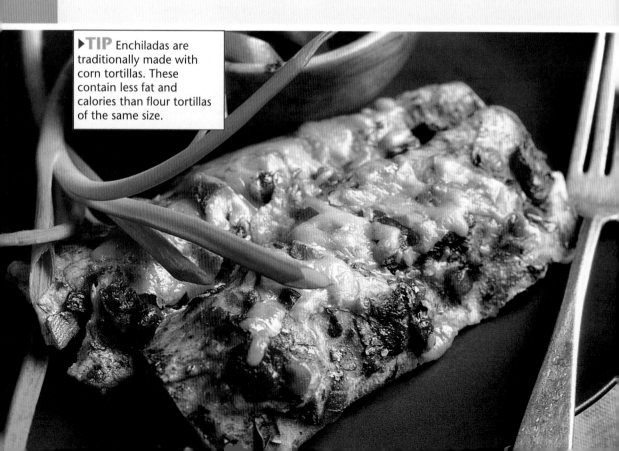

▸**TIP** Enchiladas are traditionally made with corn tortillas. These contain less fat and calories than flour tortillas of the same size.

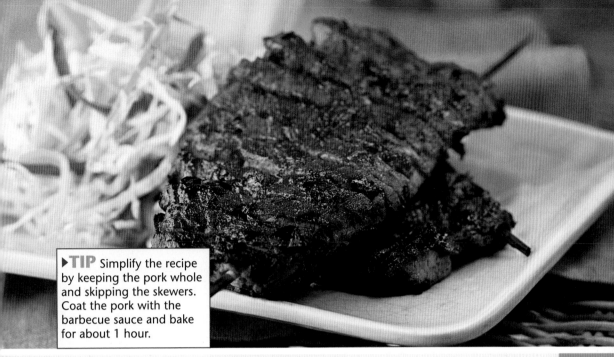

> **▶TIP** Simplify the recipe by keeping the pork whole and skipping the skewers. Coat the pork with the barbecue sauce and bake for about 1 hour.

Barbecued pork 'ribs'

SERVES 6

Meat doesn't get much fattier than pork ribs, but you can enjoy the same flavour by substituting much leaner pork fillet. You'll cut fat calories by 90 per cent.

2 pork fillets, about 350g (12oz) each, trimmed of all visible fat

1 red onion, chopped

1 red pepper, deseeded and chopped

3 garlic cloves, crushed

225ml (8fl oz) tomato ketchup

125ml (4fl oz) tomato-chilli sauce

4 tablespoons molasses or dark treacle

3 tablespoons Worcestershire sauce

2 tablespoons light soft brown sugar

2 teaspoons mild chilli powder

2 teaspoons mustard powder

Tabasco sauce to taste

1. Soak four 30–38cm (12–15in) wooden skewers in water for 30 minutes. Butterfly the pork, then cut into 'ribs' and thread onto the skewers. Cover and refrigerate.

2. Preheat the oven to 230°C (450°F, gas mark 8). Lightly spray a shallow baking tin with cooking spray. Spread the vegetables in the tin and lightly spray with cooking spray. Roast, tossing frequently, for about 15 minutes or until brown and tender.

3. Transfer to a food processor. Add the ketchup, chilli sauce, molasses, Worcestershire sauce, sugar, chilli powder, mustard and Tabasco, and purée until quite smooth. Pour into a saucepan, cover and cook for about 15 minutes, stirring occasionally. Remove 225ml (8fl oz) of the sauce for basting; keep the remaining sauce hot.

4. Heat the grill to high (or light the barbecue). Spray the grill rack generously with cooking spray. Baste both sides of the pork with sauce, then grill, turning and basting every 4 minutes, for a total of 15 minutes or until cooked through. Serve with the remaining sauce.

DISASTER FOOD	MASTER FOOD
Pork ribs	Pork fillet
115g (4oz) butter or oil	No butter or oil
100g (3½oz) brown sugar	2 tablespoons brown sugar
Kcal per serving: 665	Kcal per serving: 265
Fat per serving: 45g	Fat per serving: 5g

master your disaster foods

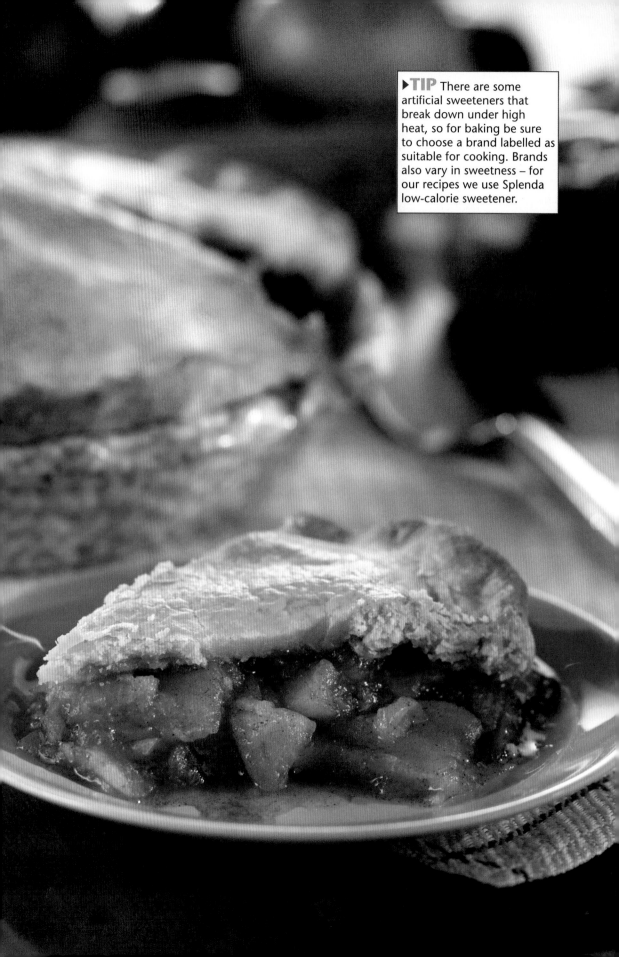

▶TIP There are some artificial sweeteners that break down under high heat, so for baking be sure to choose a brand labelled as suitable for cooking. Brands also vary in sweetness – for our recipes we use Splenda low-calorie sweetener.

Apple pie

The quintessential fruit pie doesn't have to be quintessentially fattening. This version has all the tart sweetness of the family favourite but only a third of the calories. Reduced-fat spread contains more water than butter or margarine, so work quickly when rolling out the dough to prevent the spread from becoming too soft and making the dough sticky.

40g (1½oz) reduced-fat spread for baking

70g (2½oz) plain flour

¼ teaspoon salt

1 tablespoon vegetable oil

1 tablespoon cold water

1 tablespoon rice flour or cornflour

6 medium dessert apples (such as Granny Smith), peeled, cored and sliced

4 tablespoons Splenda sweetener

½–1 tablespoon ground cinnamon

1 teaspoon skimmed milk (optional)

1. Chill the spread in the freezer until very cold but not frozen. Preheat the oven to 180°C (350°F, gas mark 4).

2. Combine the flour and salt in a medium bowl. Cut in the chilled spread with two knives until the mixture resembles coarse crumbs. Add the oil and blend quickly. Sprinkle over the water and stir lightly with a fork until moistened.

3. Shape the dough into a ball. Roll out between two sheets of lightly floured greaseproof paper to make a 23cm (9in) circle about 3mm (⅛in) thick.

4. Sprinkle the rice flour over the bottom of an 18–20cm (7–8in) pie dish (to absorb juices from the apples during cooking). Add the apples and sweetener and sprinkle with the cinnamon. Place the pastry over the apples. Crimp the edges to seal and cut slits in the top. Brush lightly with the milk, if using. Bake for about 1 hour or until the pastry is golden and the apples are tender (test through a slit).

DISASTER FOOD	MASTER FOOD
Thick pastry	Thin pastry
140g (5oz) sugar	2 tablespoons sugar substitute and ½–1 tablespoon cinnamon
175g (6oz) butter	40g (1½oz) reduced-fat spread and 1 tablespoon vegetable oil
Kcal per serving: 331	Kcal per serving: 108
Fat per serving: 19g	Fat per serving: 5g

master your disaster foods

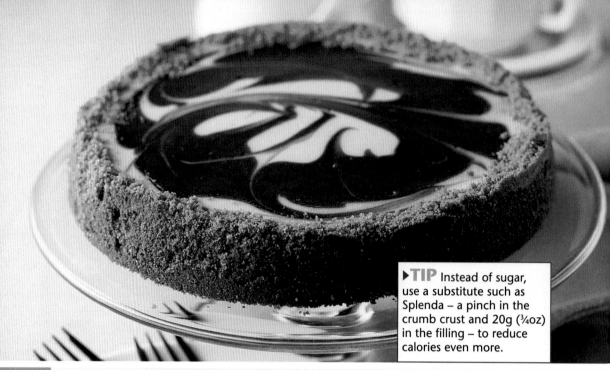

▶**TIP** Instead of sugar, use a substitute such as Splenda – a pinch in the crumb crust and 20g (¾oz) in the filling – to reduce calories even more.

Marbled cheesecake

SERVES 12

Its rich taste and creamy texture make cheesecake one of the best-loved of all desserts. Keep the romance alive by using lighter ingredients.

85g (3oz) reduced-fat digestive biscuits

50g (1¾oz) toasted wheat germ

1 tablespoon plus 200g (7oz) caster sugar

2 tablespoons light olive oil

500g (1lb 2oz) silken tofu, well drained

450g (1lb) very-low-fat soft cheese

3 tablespoons plain flour

1 extra large egg plus 2 extra large egg whites

1 teaspoon vanilla extract

4 tablespoons chocolate syrup

1. Preheat the oven to 180˚C (350˚F, gas mark 4).

2. Combine the digestive biscuits, wheat germ and 1 tablespoon of the sugar in a food processor and process into fine crumbs. Add the oil and process until moistened. Press the mixture over the bottom and partway up the sides of a 23cm (9in) springform tin. Bake for about 10 minutes or until set. Cool.

3. Put the tofu, soft cheese, flour, egg and egg whites, vanilla and the remaining sugar into the food processor and process until smooth.

4. Measure 225ml (8fl oz) of the tofu mixture into a small bowl and stir in the chocolate syrup. Pour the remaining mixture into the crumb crust. Pour the chocolate mixture in a ring on top and swirl in with a knife to marble. Bake for 45 minutes. Turn off the oven and leave the cheesecake inside for 45 minutes. Cool to room temperature before chilling overnight.

DISASTER FOOD	MASTER FOOD
225g (8oz) full-fat soft cheese	450g (1lb) very-low-fat soft cheese
450ml (16fl oz) soured cream	500g tofu
2 whole eggs	1 whole egg and 2 egg whites
Butter in crumb crust	Olive oil in crumb crust
Kcal per serving: 340	Kcal per serving: 241
Fat per serving: 21g	Fat per serving: 8g

Chocolate mousse

SERVES 4

Who would guess that you could have the luscious flavour and smooth, rich texture of this popular dessert with a fraction of the usual fat and calories? But you can, thanks to no-added-sugar pudding mix and semi-skimmed milk.

300ml (½ pint) semi-skimmed milk

1 packet no-added-sugar chocolate instant pudding mix

125ml (4fl oz) whipping cream, whipped until thick

1. Pour the milk into a medium bowl and add the pudding mix. Stir until dissolved.

2. Fold in the whipped cream. Cover and chill for at least 30 minutes, but serve within 2 hours.

DISASTER FOOD	MASTER FOOD
450ml (16fl oz) double cream	300ml (½ pint) semi-skimmed milk with whipping cream
115g (4oz) chocolate plus 150g (5½oz) sugar	No-added-sugar chocolate pudding mix
4 eggs	No eggs
Kcal per serving: 942	Kcal per serving: 211
Fat per serving: 75g	Fat per serving: 16g

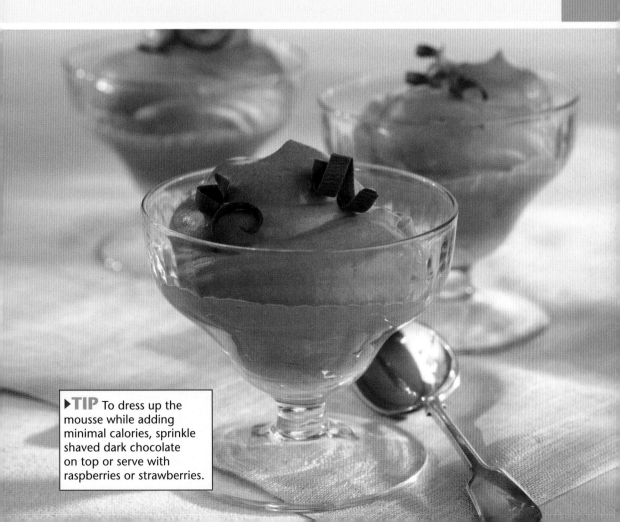

▶**TIP** To dress up the mousse while adding minimal calories, sprinkle shaved dark chocolate on top or serve with raspberries or strawberries.

STEP 5 Sensitize with exercise

The Plate Approach will take you a long way towards slimming your waistline, lowering your blood sugar and possibly even getting you off diabetes medication or reducing your dosage. But there is more you can do. Taking exercise is another way in which you can trim fat from your body and control your condition. Physical activity achieves the same result naturally as some drugs: it sensitizes the body's cells to insulin so that they soak up more glucose from the bloodstream, which brings down blood sugar levels.

In this step, you'll discover a simple plan to introduce more exercise in your life, 5 minutes at a time.

We will also provide you with an easy, 10-minute muscle-building workout to boost your metabolism and a relaxing routine to help you to wind down at the end of the day. You'll discover how simple activities – from doing housework to tensing your muscles while you sit in your car – can help to tone your muscles, burn calories and bring your blood sugar levels closer to normal.

Exercise can make or break your efforts to lose weight and control your blood sugar. The DO IT study – and a long list of other studies over the years – have proved this. In one study comparing weight-loss programmes using either diet alone, exercise alone or a combination of both, people who combined approaches lost the most weight after a year. A year after that, those who both ate less and exercised more were still ahead of the diet-only people, who regained much of their weight.

It is easy to see why exercise is so important. Let's say you wanted to cut 500kcal (calories) a day – about the amount needed to lose 500g (1lb 2oz) a week. You could consume 500 fewer kcal, but if you burned half of those by being more active, you'd have to cut only 250kcal from your diet. That would make your eating plan seem far less stringent.

Exercise also increases your metabolism, so your body uses up more calories even when you are not active. Think of exercising as adding booster rockets to the slow burn of weight loss.

For people with diabetes, though, exercise does much more than aid weight loss. It also sensitizes cells to insulin – in effect, reversing the insulin resistance that characterizes Type 2 diabetes. How does it do this? When you work your muscles, they become more efficient at using glucose. That is because active muscles demand more energy (in the form of glucose), which forces them to squeeze more glucose out of the blood. This glucose-gobbling effect continues even after you have stopped exercising, lowering your blood sugar for hours after a workout. As your body becomes more conditioned, your toned muscles require more energy all the time, making the glucose-controlling effects of exercise virtually permanent, as long as you stay active. What's more, physical activity also reduces your risk of problems common among people with diabetes, such as high blood pressure, heart attack, stroke and arthritis.

Once you get going, you'll find that exercise feels so good that you will want to keep doing it. (Remember, your body was designed to move, not to sit all day.) You'll feel more energetic,

10 ways to burn calories in 10 minutes

▸ Walking, 30-minute mile	32kcal
▸ Bowling	38kcal
▸ Ballroom dancing	38kcal
▸ Vacuuming	45kcal
▸ Cycling, 10 miles an hour	51kcal
▸ Water aerobics	51kcal
▸ Weeding or digging in the garden	57kcal
▸ Playing tennis (doubles)	77kcal
▸ Horseback riding (trot)	83kcal
▸ Swimming (moderate effort)	89kcal

sleep better, and even look better. So how do you start? With Action One, a simple plan to increase the time you spend walking. That's because when we say 'exercise', the sort of activity we're talking about is taking an evening walk around your neighbourhood, following a circuit through the local park or going window shopping at your nearest shopping centre. We will ask that you dedicate a certain amount of time on most days to walking – starting with just 10 minutes and adding 5 minutes a week. But you should also take every opportunity to put one foot in front of the other wherever you go.

Once you have got into the swing of walking, it will be time to start toning your muscles even more with our simple Sugar-Buster routine. It takes only 10 minutes – and don't forget that by working your muscles you help to reverse your insulin resistance.

Exercise needn't be restricted to the times when you are 'exercising'. You can exercise while you are waiting in the car at a red light, queuing at the post office – or even brushing your teeth. Your day is filled with countless opportunites to fit in quick exercises that tone your muscles and help to bring down your blood sugar. Our 30-second Fitness Boosters will help you to make the most of idle time that you would otherwise waste.

Another reason to move your body is to release tension and calm your mind. As you will learn in Step Six, relaxing is an important way to keep blood sugar under control. That is

Exercise and hypoglycaemia

Exercise is so effective in bringing down your blood sugar that you need to make sure that it doesn't drop too low and cause hypoglycaemia (see page 15). You should time exercise to fit in with your medication or insulin schedule (see page 54), but also be prepared to deal with hypoglycaemia if it occurs.

- **Know the signs** Confusion, shaking, lightheadedness or difficulty speaking all indicate that you should stop exercising immediately.
- **Have a snack handy** When blood sugar is too low, you can quickly bring it back up with a high-carbohydrate snack, such as a couple of glucose tablets, a square of chocolate or a glass of non-diet soft drink or juice.
- **Use the buddy system** Try to walk or work out with someone who could lend a hand in an emergency.
- **Carry identification** Even if you're just strolling through your neighbourhood, carry ID with your name, address and phone number, plus emergency information such as how to reach your doctor and the dosages of your medication or insulin.

because stress hormones directly raise blood sugar – and contribute to weight gain. Our 10-minute yoga-based programme of simple, soothing movements will unclench your muscles and help to rid your body and mind of stress. We suggest that you use it to wind down at the end of the day, but you can do it in the morning or any other time you wish.

Remember to check with your doctor before starting any exercise programme, especially if you are aged over 35, have had diabetes for more than 10 years or already show signs of heart disease, poor circulation or nerve damage. Most people, however, should have no problem with the exercises in this chapter, especially if they start gradually.

ACTION 1 Get walking with our simple exercise plan

Walking belongs at the core of your activity plan because it's an ideal way to get your body moving. Studies find that walking lowers blood sugar even more effectively than other forms of exercise, partly because it engages your muscles for sustained periods of time, which keeps demand for blood glucose high. Just as important, walking is an easy activity that requires no special skills or equipment. You can do it any time, anywhere.

It's true that committing yourself to walking on a regular basis means that you will need to make an investment of time. In the Forward by Five walking plan your goal is to walk at least five days a week. Impossible? Some of the people in the DO IT study thought the same thing – until the pounds started dropping off and exercise became a priority. You won't get to that point instantly, and we are not asking you to. Instead, you will build up walking time gradually, in the following way.

START WITH 10 MINUTES

That's about the time it takes to walk a single loop around the block – or to make a pot of coffee, browse through a magazine or check the TV listings for the week ahead. In other words, anyone can manage to carve out 10 minutes from a day, yet that is all you need to start with.

For five days during the first week, do your 10-minute walks. Once you get going, you'll be surprised how quickly your walks become a habit. That's not as glib as it may sound. We realize that the simple act of going outside to take some exercise may seem like a big change. In fact, the hardest part may be taking that first step out of the door, so start with that. Open the door and step outside as if you were getting the morning paper. Next, walk to the end of the driveway. Then head to the end of the street, as if you had seen a neighbour you want to talk to. Keep moving in small stages like that, and you will have walked for 10 minutes in no time.

The next thing you know, you may even start to look forward to getting out. Think of all that awaits you: fresh air, time away from your responsibilities and a chance to see what's going on in the neighbourhood (you'll notice plenty of things you would have overlooked driving by in a car).

MOVE **FORWARD BY 5** MINUTES EACH WEEK

Five more minutes a day is not a lot to ask, and it may not seem like a big improvement in the amount of exercise you do. In fact, that's the point. By adding just 5 minutes each week, you'll increase your walking almost imperceptibly, so it never seems like a big deal. Yet those minutes add up and can make a significant impact on your blood sugar. After all, 5 more minutes on five days amounts to 25 minutes of extra walking time per week.

Pick an official starting day for your walking week – most people choose Sunday or Monday – and add on 5 minutes of walking that day, then try to stick to your new routine until you move forward by another 5 minutes. Aim to build up to at least 45 minutes a day. If you start with 10 minutes and stay on track, that will take you eight weeks. Even before you reach that target, though, you will trim weight from your body, and maintaining that routine will ensure that the pounds stay off. If you want to continue improving after your eight weeks are up, increase the intensity by walking faster or more often.

TAKE TIME TO REASSESS

One day a week, preferably in the middle of your weekly walking cycle, you should take time to assess yourself. Your physical condition and capabilities are different from

Steps to success

Maria Holland, a 34-year-old participant in the DO IT study, remembers the moment she realized what exercise could do to bring down her blood sugar levels. 'One night after dinner, I tested my blood sugar and it was 12.4mmol/l,' she says. 'Then I went for a 20-minute walk and took a reading again, and my sugars were down to 7.4mmol/l. I'd never done a before-and-after comparison before, and it was a real eye-opener to see how big a difference I could make just by walking.'

That was incentive enough to make 20-minute walks part of her routine just about every day. 'I felt that I could start with 20 minutes,' she says. 'I was capable of exercise, but until then, I just didn't do it.' Two weeks into her walking routine, however, she started to feel a definite change of attitude. 'Exercise is one of those things you don't always feel like doing, but if you do it anyway, you feel good afterwards,' says Marie. 'I started to feel that I wanted to do more.' By the third or fourth week, 'I became almost addicted to it,' she says. 'If I didn't go out for a walk, it just felt wrong.' Marie quickly worked up to 30-minute walks and would even go as long as an hour if she had the time. Blessed with a safe neighbourhood, she would often take peaceful, quiet walks through residential streets at night.

Just as important, Marie started finding ways to work more steps into her day. At the hospital where she worked as a nurse, for example, she would take the stairs instead of the lift if she had to climb three flights or less. At home, she took over the task of mowing the lawn from her husband. And whenever she took one of her children, aged 14, 12 and 3, to football practice, she would walk the perimeter of the field instead of sitting and waiting.

Within two months, Marie's blood sugar dropped to normal levels – something that medication had been unable to accomplish before she exercised – and she shed 30kg (4st 9lb) during the study. Since then, she has lost a further 13.6kg (2st 2lb). Part of the secret, she says, is that walking helps her to stick to her eating plan. 'If I eat a cupcake, I think of all the exercise it would take to burn it off,' she says. 'It's a mindset you get into that keeps you motivated.'

everybody else's, so this is an opportunity for you to decide whether or not you should make any adjustments to your walking programme. Ask yourself the following questions.

- Is it hard to get motivated to walk because the effort seems daunting?
- Do I feel tired after I finish a walk?
- Does walking cause any kind of pain?
- Do I feel invigorated and full of energy?
- Does the amount I'm walking seem tame?
- Am I free from uncomfortable soreness or any damage to my feet?

If you answer yes to any of the first three questions, especially if you are clinically obese, trim today's walk back by 5 minutes. If exercise feels punishing, you are not likely to persevere with it, so don't feel you have to push yourself beyond what you – or your body – are ready for. Perhaps you are just feeling tired today. Tomorrow, go back to this week's walking time. If you still feel fatigued and sluggish then stick with 5 fewer minutes for the rest of this week. When you feel comfortable about adding another 5 minutes, proceed with the plan.

If you answer yes to any of the last three questions, add another 5 minutes to your walk today: you are clearly capable of more, and this is a chance to push yourself. Tomorrow, either stick with the new time goal or revert to the week's original plan – the choice is yours.

BUILD IN **WILD CARD** DAYS

Our programme calls for you to walk five days a week. So what do you do on the other two days? Anything but nothing. Don't think of 'off' days as holidays from activity. Instead, think of them as Wild Card days, when anything goes – as long as your body is being active in some way. If you want to do some more walking, go ahead. You may prefer to skip the walking and work up a sweat in your garden instead. Or you might choose to kick a ball with your child or grandchild for 20 minutes and then walk home from the playground as your exercise for the day. Wild Card days are also perfect for hobbies such as golf or tennis (and provide an opportunity to take up a new hobby, such as ballroom dancing).

STEP UP YOUR EFFORTS

Don't think of your walks as the only movement you need to do all day. In the not so distant past people walked almost everywhere they needed to go, and daily life is still filled with opportunities to power yourself to your destination, whether it's the second floor of a shopping centre (take the stairs, not the escalators) or a newsagent down the street. Every step you take, whether or not you're consciously exercising, burns calories. You should consciously aim to take more of them, even when you're not on one of your walks.

Here's one way to do it. When your regular walking hits the 30-minute mark, buy a pedometer, a small device you wear on your waist that counts each step you take. The number of steps you take in a given amount of time varies according to the length of your stride, but your numbers will already be well into the thousands if you are walking 30 minutes a day. Build on that by trying to hit a higher mark. If you've walked 8,500 steps a day, for example, aim for 9,000. Work towards the goal of 10,000 steps a day. Even if you're not counting, take every chance to walk more.

If you have spent your life looking for ways to save steps, it may be hard to reverse your mental conditioning and think of ways to become less efficient. But those small losses in efficiency add up to gains that will speed your efforts to control your blood sugar – and there's nothing inefficient about that. Here are seven ways to step up your efforts.

- If you are meeting a friend, catch up over a stroll instead of a cup of coffee.
- If you have a mobile, walk while you talk. They don't call them mobile phones for nothing.

Help!

I know exercise helps me, but I can't get motivated to go out for a walk.

Call it the threshold barrier. Taking that first step is always the hardest. Sometimes, with life so busy, you don't even think about exercise. At other times, you know you should but lack the willpower. Here are some steps that can help.

- Put your walking shoes by the door at night so you will see them first thing in the morning. They will remind you that getting out there is a priority.

- Have a destination in mind. Going to the shop, post office, newsagent or café makes walking seem more purposeful and time-worthy.

- Book walking time on your calendar. Once you have booked the time, stick adhesive reminder notes on the fridge and doors to spur you on – a technique shown to work in studies.

- Enlist a friend to walk with you or, if that's not possible, to call and ask if you have walked. A sense of accountability is one of the best motivators for exercise.

- Find an article of clothing that fitted you when you weighed 10 per cent less or a photo of yourself at the time. Display it prominently as an inspirational reminder of your goal.

- During TV commercials, walk on the spot, go up and down the stairs, or walk round the perimeter of the house.
- If you have a local errand to do, walk there and back instead of taking the car.
- Don't fight for a parking space near the entrance of a car park. Instead park at the far end of the car park and walk.
- At the supermarket, return your shopping trolley to the front of the store instead of leaving it in the car park.
- In airports, walk around the terminal while waiting for your flight, and avoid the moving travelators.

ACTION 2 Tone your muscles with our Sugar-Buster routine

Walking is aerobic exercise. That is, it is sustained over a period of time, so it gets your heart and lungs working and builds endurance. It's a great start, but it's not the only kind of exercise you can – or should – be doing to help beat diabetes. Building strength is important, too. Why bother building stronger muscles? The reason is simple. Even when you're not exercising, bigger, denser muscles need more energy, which means they burn more calories and siphon more glucose out of your blood. So you can beat diabetes simply by sitting still – as long as you keep your muscles in shape.

The investment you need to make to get those results may not be as great as you think. The routine that we have designed, on pages 144-151, can be done in 10 minutes – roughly the time you'd spend watching commercials during a typical hour-long TV show – so you can do this workout during your favourite programme. If you have never done strength exercises before (or simply don't enjoy them very much), we have broken the workout down into 2 or 3-minute sequences that don't have to be done at the same time. Consider the advantages of exercising in 2-minute sequences.

- You can fit strength exercise into any schedule. For example, you can do one sequence in the morning, another at noon and the third in the late afternoon. You can do one sequence on different days of the week so you develop a habit of doing a little exercise almost every day. Or, of course, you can do the entire workout in a single session.

Walking is one of the safest forms of exercise, but when you have diabetes, complications such as nerve damage and impaired circulation can put your feet at risk of serious damage. You should not avoid walking, but you should take the following precautions to keep your feet healthy.

▸ Check your feet every day. If you have nerve damage, you could have sores, cuts, swelling or infection that you can't feel.

▸ Avoid cracked skin and reduce the risk of infection by towelling your feet off thoroughly after bathing, especially between your toes. Rub lotion or cream on the tops and bottoms of your feet to keep them moist, and sprinkle talcum powder between your toes to prevent fungal growth.

▸ Trim your toenails at least once a week after bathing, cutting straight across the nails and smoothing them with a nail file or emery board.

▸ Always wear socks and shoes. Socks should be seamless to avoid pressure points and friction, and shoes are best made of leather, which moulds to your feet and breathes to keep them drier.

▸ To boost blood circulation to your feet, wiggle your toes for 5 minutes two or three times a day. Avoid tight elastic socks, don't cross your legs for long periods of time and put your feet up when you're sitting.

● You never exercise so hard that you work up a sweat, so you can do the exercises at any time and wearing any type of clothing.

● You can squeeze exercise into small chunks of time, such as the moments between getting dressed in the morning and having breakfast, or the time between getting home from work and sitting down to your evening meal.

THE **SUGAR-BUSTER** ROUTINE

Both efficient and effective, this workout uses exercises that work more than one major muscle group at once, saving you time and effort. Some exercises (such as the Slow hundred) draw on the torso-strengthening methods of Pilates, while others (such as the Airplane pose) are adapted from yoga. All are basic exercises that will come easily to people at any level of ability. Here are some guidelines to get you started.

STICK TO SEQUENCES The routine is divided into three sequences. Do just one sequence if you're short of time or energy, or do the whole routine in a single session.

- **Upper body** works the chest, triceps and shoulders.
- **Lower body** targets the hamstrings and quadriceps.
- **Core body** strengthens the abdominals and lower back.

Sample activity schedule

Here's an example of how the Forward by Five walking plan might be put into practice over the course of eight weeks. Remember, if you find the plan too easy, add more minutes. Use your Wild Card days to substitute any physical activity you want, from playing ball with the children to raking up garden leaves, for

	WEEK 1 GET OUTSIDE	WEEK 2 BUILD ON YOUR NEW HABIT	WEEK 3 TAKE YOURSELF TO A NEW DESTINATION	WEEK 4 EASE INTO THE SUGAR-BUSTER ROUTINE
MON	10-minute walk	15-minute walk	20-minute walk	25-minute walk Sugar Buster: upper body
TUES	10-minute walk	15-minute walk	20-minute walk	25-minute walk
WED	Assessment day: 5 or 15-minute walk	Assessment day: 10 or 20-minute walk	Assessment day: 15 or 25-minute walk	Assessment day: 20 or 30-minute walk
THUR	10-minute walk	15-minute walk	20-minute walk	25-minute walk Sugar Buster: lower body
FRI	*Wild Card day*	*Wild Card day*	*Wild Card day*	*Wild Card day*
SAT	10-minute walk	15-minute walk	20-minute walk	25-minute walk Sugar Buster: core body
SUN	*Wild Card day*	*Wild Card day*	*Wild Card day*	*Wild Card day*

ESTABLISH A SCHEDULE Introduce the exercises gradually (one a day is a good start), but you should aim eventually to do the entire programme at least twice a week. Do the whole workout on two different days, or do one sequence a day.

walking. We have also suggested how you might fit in your Sugar-Buster routine. You can swap the days' activities around, but be sure to decide on a schedule *before* you start, then post it on your refrigerator or write it in your calendar. Committing to a schedule greatly increases your chances of sticking to the plan.

	WEEK 5 KEEP ON GOING	WEEK 6 COMBINE THE SUGAR-BUSTER SEGMENTS	WEEK 7 YOUR BODY IS LOOKING BETTER	WEEK 8 BRAVO! NOW KEEP UP THE GOOD WORK
MON	30-minute walk Sugar Buster: upper body	35-minute walk Sugar-Buster routine	40-minute walk Sugar-Buster routine	45-minute walk Sugar-Buster routine
TUES	30-minute walk	35-minute walk	40-minute walk	45-minute walk
WED	Assessment day: 25 or 35-minute walk	Assessment day: 30 or 40-minute walk	Assessment day: 35 or 45-minute walk	Assessment day: 40 or 50-minute walk
THUR	30-minute walk Sugar Buster: lower body	35-minute walk Sugar-Buster routine	40-minute walk Sugar-Buster routine	45-minute walk Sugar-Buster routine
FRI	*Wild Card day*	*Wild Card day*	*Wild Card day*	*Wild Card day*
SAT	30-minute walk Sugar Buster: core body	35-minute walk Sugar-Buster routine	40-minute walk Sugar-Buster Routine	45-minute walk Sugar-Buster routine
SUN	*Wild Card day*	*Wild Card day*	*Wild Card day*	*Wild Card day*

3 Include stealthy exercises

ACTION

What kind of exercise can you do while you are waiting in a check-out queue at the supermarket? The kind you can do with a smile on your face – because if people realized you were working your buttock muscles, they might find you more interesting than the tabloid headlines. Our 30-second Fitness Boosters, on pages 152-161, will not only build your body, they will also keep your thoughts occupied – not a bad thing if you would otherwise be thinking how delicious a chocolate bar from the checkout rack would taste right now.

Most of us hate to kill time, and yet we face countless opportunities during the day to do just that. From now on, be alert for those small moments of idle time during your day and look forward to them with anticipation, because they are the perfect opportunity to build some extra exercise into your day. You can do some of the 30-second Fitness Boosters while queuing at the bank, sitting in a traffic jam or waiting for friends or family members to turn up at an agreed meeting place. Others you can do in the privacy of your home while

How to burn calories without noticing

1. Take the escalator, but climb the stairs while you ride. You'll get there faster and use your muscles while you're at it. Just 5 minutes of stair climbing burns 144kcal.

2. Instead of trying to carry lots of bags or other items upstairs all at once, take them one at a time.

3. While you are waiting in a doctor's surgery, on a train platform or at an airport, stay on your feet. Standing burns 36 more kcal per hour than sitting.

4. Rake up garden leaves instead of using a leaf blower. You'll burn 50 more kcal every half-hour.

5. Scrub your floors more often. Putting some elbow grease into cleaning floors is more intense exercise than vacuuming – and it makes your floors look better, too.

6. Chew sugarless gum. Research has found that the action of jaw muscles alone burns about 11kcal an hour.

7. Wash your car by hand instead of taking it through the automatic carwash. You'll burn an extra 280kcal in an hour.

8. Play with the children. Impromptu games of Frisbee, football or tag – or just throwing and catching a ball – will help you to use energy and set a good example for your children. You'll burn 80-137kcal for every 10 minutes of activity.

Quiz
Analysing your activity

It's all too easy to allow false assumptions or lack of time to get in the way of being more active. Find out if any obstacles are preventing you from taking exercise, and how to deal with them, by answering the following questions.

1. **Tick each statement about lifestyle that is true for you:**
- ❑ I do work such as pushing a lawnmower or gardening for at least an hour a week.
- ❑ I do moderately vigorous housework such as scrubbing the floor or cleaning windows for a total of at least an hour a week.
- ❑ I make a habit of using the stairs instead of the lift.
- ❑ In my job I often walk or move around.

2. **Tick each statement about exercise that is true for you:**
- ❑ I walk, play tennis or ride a bike for at least 40 minutes a week.
- ❑ I walk once in a while.
- ❑ The only exercise I get is looking for the remote control.

3. **The best exercise for losing weight is:**
- ❑ Running.
- ❑ Walking.
- ❑ Swimming.
- ❑ Cycling.

4. **Which of the following do you think will burn more calories?**
- ❑ Walking round the neighbourhood for 10 minutes after breakfast and 10 minutes after dinner.
- ❑ Strolling an extra 2 minutes to and from your car on five trips to the supermarket.
- ❑ Walking 20 minutes down the high street.

5. **Tick any of the following statements that reflect your feelings or beliefs:**
- ❑ Exercise will just make me hungry, and I'll eat more.
- ❑ I don't like to sweat.
- ❑ I have no energy for exercise.
- ❑ I'm just not an exercise person.

6. **When I'm feeling tired, I:**
- ❑ Flop down in front of the TV.
- ❑ Reach for a chocolate bar.
- ❑ Take a brisk 10-minute walk.

7. **For each amount of time, list an activity you normally do each day that you could eliminate without major consequences:**

3 minutes: _____

_____

10 minutes: _____

_____

20 minutes: _____

_____

30 minutes: _____

_____

8. **My favourite physical activities are:**
- ❑ Playing badminton or Frisbee, or throwing a ball.
- ❑ Walking my dog.
- ❑ Doing the housework.
- ❑ Shopping.
- ❑ Other. _____

_____

_____

Turn the page to evaluate your answers.

Quiz
What your score means

1. If you ticked any of these answers, great! You're already working physical activity into every week. But don't rest on your laurels: several of these would need to be true to have an effect on your weight. Our exercise programme will help you to build more movement into your life – which is especially important if you didn't tick any answers here.

2. If you ticked the first answer, congratulations. You're well on your way to getting in shape, which will increase your life expectancy. If you ticked the second answer, it must mean you like walking, so you'll do fine on the Forward by Five walking plan. If you ticked the third answer, pay special attention to the advice in Step Five: it will get you going again.

3. These all help you to lose weight, but only if you persevere with them. Since studies find that people are more likely to stick with walking than with other exercise routines, we have made walking the basis of our Forward by Five Walking Plan.

4. All of these burn the same number of calories, which shows how easy it is to work more activity into your life, regardless of your schedule.

5. If you didn't tick any boxes, great! If you did, don't let excuses like these stop you from exercising. Studies show that moderate exercise does not stimulate your appetite. None of the exercises in our programme are so intense that you'll sweat a lot. Moving your body will boost your energy, not drain it. And you don't have to be an 'exercise person', you simply have to be more active.

6. Flopping down on the sofa won't do much to help, but the walk will. A brisk 10-minute walk can give you more energy than eating a chocolate bar – a 1997 study proved it. Exercise boosts a hormone that increases energy. In Step Five, you'll find plenty of ways to fit quick bursts of activity into your day.

7. If you have 3 minutes to spare you can do one of the sequences from our Sugar-Buster routine. If you have 10 minutes you can do the whole routine or the Day's-end wind-down. If you have 30 minutes that's plenty of time for a walk on the Forward by Five walking plan.

8. The cardinal rule for making your life more active is to do what you like. Find a physical activity that you enjoy, then do it more often.

you go about your normal everyday activities such as brushing your teeth or waiting for the kettle of water to boil for tea.

ACTION 4 Do the Day's-end wind-down

After a long day, doing more exercise may be the last thing on your mind. But our yoga-based routine isn't so much about exercise as about stretching and relaxing or refreshing. It's perfect for either evening or morning. Yoga is famous for relieving stress, promoting health and making muscles more flexible – an element of fitness that is frequently overlooked but essential for increasing mobility, relieving stiffness and promoting a sense of well-being. This routine, on pages 162-171, may even help to keep your blood sugar down and dampen the rise in glucose that many people with diabetes experience in the morning. How is this achieved? By lowering your levels of stress hormones. (You'll find out more about this in Step Six.)

You don't have to study with a guru or even take a class to begin putting yoga-based moves into practice. The poses and movements in the Day's-end wind-down routine are simple. Perform them in the order we have suggested so that each exercise leads straight into the next. Once you become familiar with the routine, don't pause between movements; just let the entire workout flow until you reach the end, which should take only about 10 minutes. Don't be in a rush to finish, though: the idea is to get off life's roller coaster and relax.

While moving through the exercises, breathe evenly and deliberately and coordinate your movements with your breathing (we'll tell you when to breathe in and out). The more automatic the routine becomes, the easier it will be to let your mind go, which is an important part of relaxing.

If you're like many people, you may discover that you are not very flexible. Take heart: the more often you do this routine, the more flexible you will become.

Y ou can perform the entire Sugar-Buster routine in about 10 minutes, so there are no excuses for not fitting it in. To make strength training even easier, you can do only the upper body sequence, the lower body sequence or the core body sequence, then do a different sequence tomorrow. Each of them takes just 3 minutes.

▶ Upper body

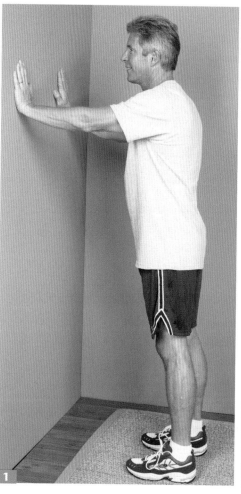 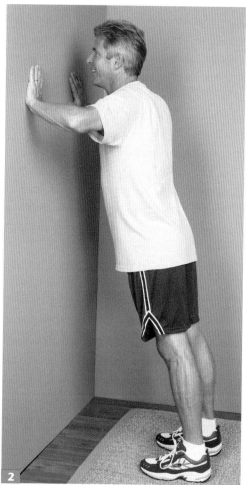

Wall push

Stand facing a wall about an arm's length away, with your feet directly under your hips. Lean forward and place your palms against the wall with your elbows slightly bent. Keep your shoulder blades back. **1**

Inhale as you slowly bend your elbows, bringing your chest closer to the wall. Do not arch your back. **2** Exhale and slowly press back to the starting position. Keep your core tight throughout. Do this 15 times.

▶**BENEFIT** Strengthens the chest and triceps muscles in a single movement.

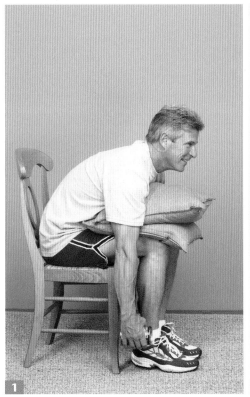
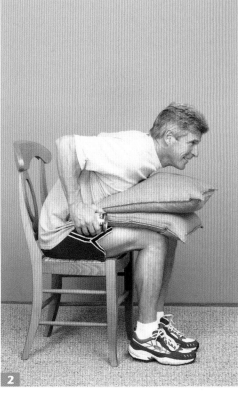

Bent-arm row

Sit on a hard-back chair with a large pillow on your lap for support. Grasping a full can of soup or a light hand weight in each hand, lean forward, keeping your back as straight as possible. Let your hands hang towards the floor, but do not allow your shoulders to drop. **1**

Exhale as you raise your elbows towards the ceiling, keeping them close to your body. **2** Hold for 1 second, then inhale as you return to the starting position. Do this 10 times.

▶**BENEFIT** Works the middle and upper back and, to a lesser extent, the biceps.

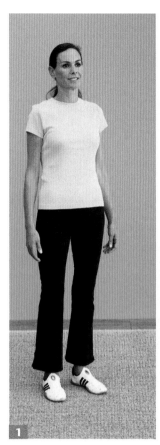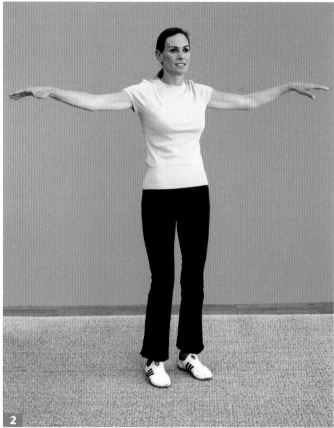

Aeroplane

Stand with your feet hip-width apart. **1** (If it's more comfortable, you can do this exercise while seated.)

Exhale and raise your arms straight out to the sides, with your palms facing down and your fingers open and relaxed, until your hands reach shoulder height. Make sure your elbows stay just below your shoulders. **2** Don't lock your elbows. Hold for 60 seconds, breathing normally, then lower your arms. Do this exercise once only.

▶**BENEFIT** Works all three sections of the shoulder muscles, which helps to maintain good upper-body posture. To increase intensity, hold a small full can of soup in each hand.

▶ Lower body

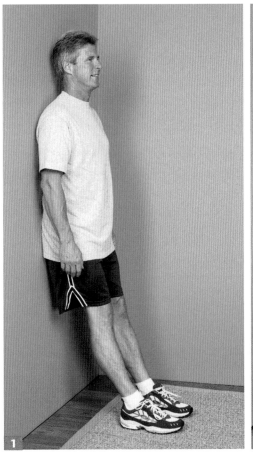 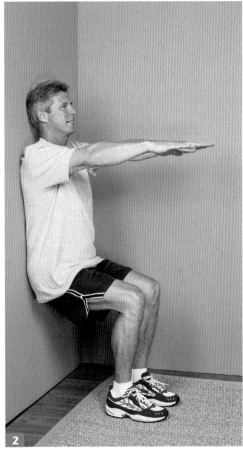

Wall slide with raised arms

Stand with your back, from your shoulders to your tailbone, pressed firmly against a wall and your feet shoulder-width apart. Keeping your back in contact with the wall, move your feet forward about 30cm (1ft). **1**

Breathe in and slide your back down the wall until your knees are bent at a 90-degree angle (or as far as is comfortable) while simultaneously raising your arms in front of you to shoulder height. **2** Hold this position for as long as is comfortable. When your legs start to feel warm, breathe in and slide back up the wall while lowering your arms to your sides. Do this four times.

▶**BENEFIT** Strengthens the shoulders and works the large muscles of the hips and buttocks for improved walking performance. To increase intensity, hold a full can of soup in each hand.

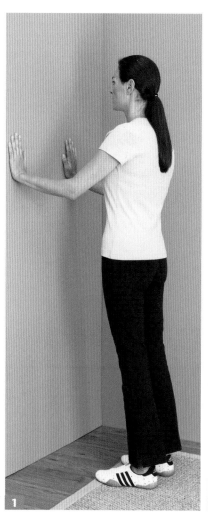
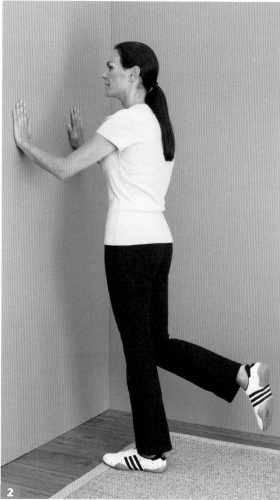

Lift pump

Stand 30cm (1ft) from a wall with your feet hip-width apart. Place your hands on the wall for support, but don't lean towards it. **1**

Exhaling, lift your right leg towards your buttocks, stopping when your knee is bent at a 90-degree angle. Do not arch your back. Keep your core tight throughout. **2** Hold for 10 seconds. Do this five times with each leg.

▶**BENEFIT** Works the hamstring muscles at the back of the upper leg. To increase intensity, put two full cans of soup in a pair of socks, tie the socks together, and drape them over the back of your ankle as you lift your leg.

▶ Core Body

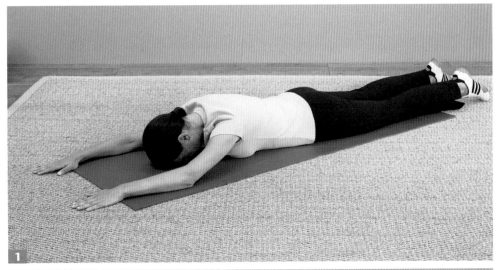

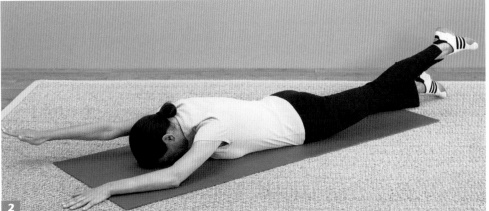

Dry swimming

Lie face down on a mat or rug with your arms and legs stretched out straight, like Superman in flight. It may be more comfortable to put a small folded towel under your forehead. **1**

Keeping your neck relaxed (don't lift your head), tense your abdominal muscles, then raise your right arm and left leg and hold for 1 second. **2** Slowly lower both limbs and repeat with the other arm and leg. Repeat for 30 seconds. Stop if you feel any back pain while doing this exercise.

▶**BENEFIT** Strengthens the lower back and bolsters the muscles that run along the lower part of the spine, improving posture and preventing lower-back pain.

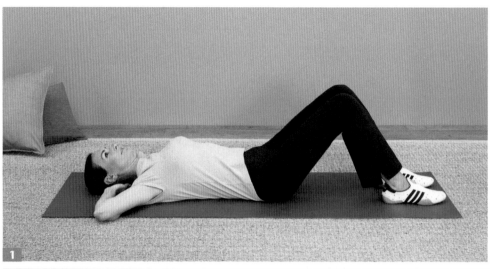

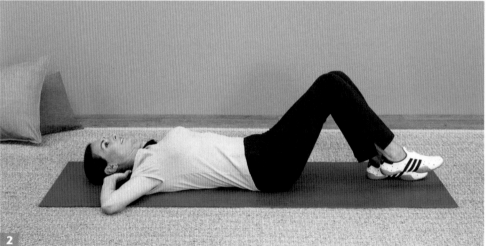

Baby lift

Lie on your back with your knees bent, your feet flat on the floor and your hands behind your head, with your elbows out to the sides. **1**

Inhale and contract your abdominal muscles so that your lower back makes contact with the floor, then raise your right foot about 3-5cm (1-2in) off the floor. **2** Hold for a count of 4 (breathing with each count: out 1, in 2, out 3, in 4), then lower your foot to the floor as you exhale. Repeat with the left leg.

▶**BENEFIT** Like traditional sit-ups, this exercise works the abdominal muscles, but it's less intense and doesn't require you to lift your head off the floor, which can strain your neck.

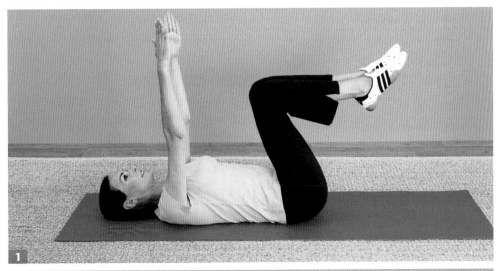

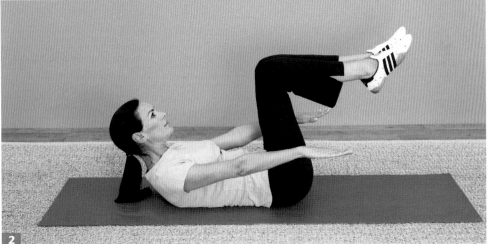

Slow hundred

Lie on your back with your legs together and your knees bent at a 90-degree angle. Inhale and raise your arms toward the ceiling without raising your shoulders off the floor. **1**

Exhaling, curl your torso up so the tops of your shoulders come off the floor. At the same time, lower your arms to your sides and hold them at hip height. **2**

Contracting your abdominal muscles, pump your arms up and down (imagine you're using a bicycle pump), counting each pump until you reach 100. Do not let your chin poke out while doing this exercise.

▶**BENEFIT** Strengthens the 'core' muscles: the abdominals, the lower-back muscles and the muscles attached to the spine.

*E*ven as you go through your usual routine, you can add more movement to your day. Do one of these 30-second Fitness Boosters while you're brushing your teeth, sitting in the car, standing in a queue, sitting at your desk or waiting for the kettle to boil.

▶ At the sink

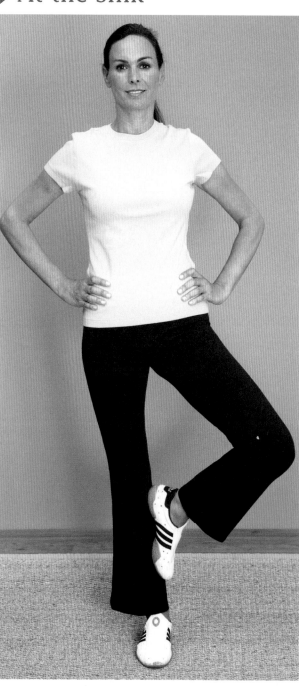

Tree pose

Stand up straight with your legs together. Slowly raise your left knee to the side, resting the bottom of your left foot against the inner calf of your right leg. Balance there for a count of 15, keeping your right knee unlocked. Pull your stomach in for support and keep your back straight and your chin up. Think about 'growing tall' through the top of your head. Repeat on the other side.

▶**BENEFIT** Strengthens the lower body and core support muscles of the lower back and abdomen.

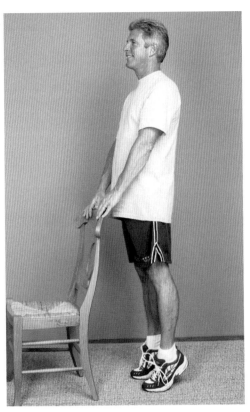

Calf raise

Stand with your feet directly under your hips, with your arms resting comfortably at your sides or your hands on the sink (or a chair) if you need help with balance. Slowly rise on your toes and hold for 30 seconds, then slowly lower yourself back down. Do this three times.

▶BENEFIT Strengthens the calves and shins, which improves agility and balance and helps you to push off with your toes when walking.

▶In the car

Steering wheel lift press

While you are waiting at a red light, grasp the bottom of the steering wheel with your palms up. Inhale and then, while exhaling, push up on the wheel with your palms as hard as you can. Hold while breathing normally until the light turns green.

▶BENEFIT Works the biceps, the primary load-bearing muscles of the arms.

Abdominal squeeze

While you are waiting at a red light or stop sign, gently breathe in and out, allowing your diaphragm to descend so that your stomach pushes out. Then don't breathe in and gently draw in your abdominal muscles as if you are trying to pull your navel back towards your spine. Hold this and breathe normally for up to 60 seconds.

▶BENEFIT Improves posture and tones the stomach to support your back and make you look slimmer.

▶ Standing in a queue

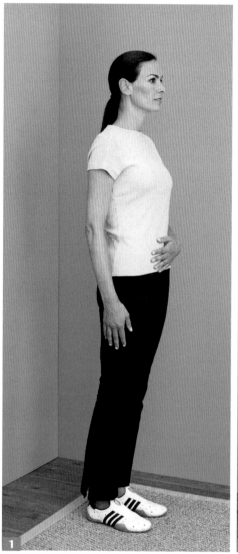 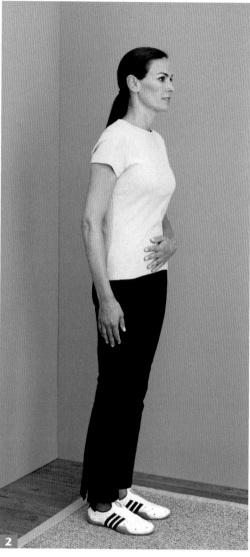

Standing abdominal squeeze

Stand with your feet hip-width apart. **1** Keeping your neck, shoulders and arms relaxed, breathe in and out. Then don't breathe in and gently pull in your stomach using your abdominal muscles, as though a belt is being tightened around your midsection. **2** Hold this and breathe normally for 60 seconds. Do this three times.

▶**BENEFIT** Doing this exercise while standing strengthens muscles that support your back against the strain of extra weight in your stomach.

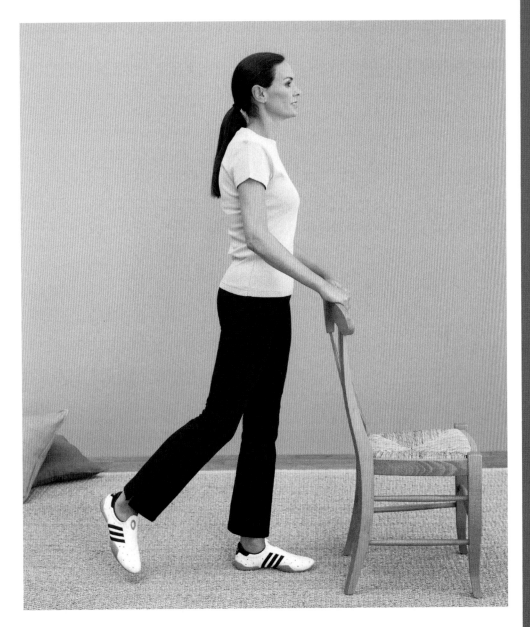

Buttock toner

Stand up straight with your feet hip-width apart, your arms at your sides (or on a chair if you need help with your balance) and your shoulders relaxed. Squeeze the muscles of your buttocks together as tightly as you can, hold in your stomach, and move your right leg about 5cm (2in) behind you with your foot off the floor. Keep your trunk upright. Do not lean forward at your shoulders or arch your back. Hold for 10 seconds, then change legs. Do at least three times with each leg.

▶BENEFIT Strengthens the humble but powerful muscles in your buttocks, which are involved in virtually every movement your body makes.

▶At your desk

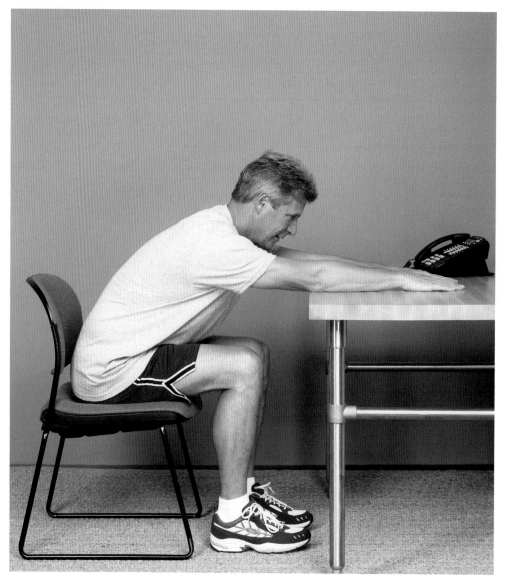

Upper back push-down

Sit at your desk, preferably in a chair without wheels. Position the chair
60-90cm (2-3ft) from the desk and keep your feet flat on the floor. Inhale
and bend forward, extending your arms straight onto the desktop with
your palms down and your fingers spread apart. Exhale and press down
with your hands and forearms as hard as you can while holding in your
abdominal muscles. Hold for 30 seconds. Do this four times.

▶**BENEFIT** Strengthens the lower body and core support muscles of the lower back
and abdomen.

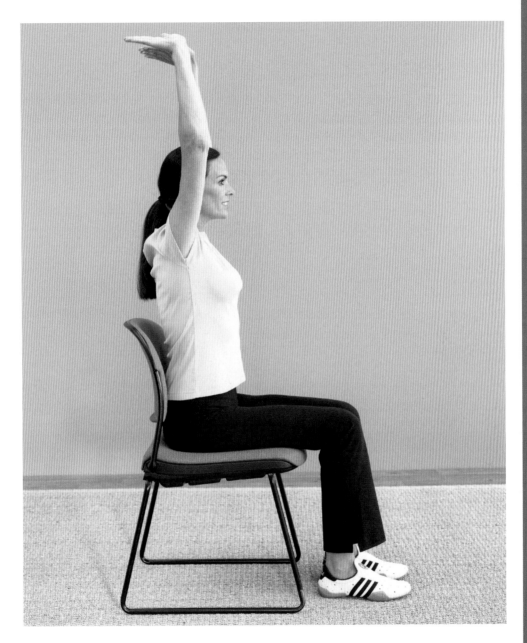

Overhead press

Sit up straight with your back firmly against the back of your chair
and your feet flat on the floor, about hip-width apart. Raise your arms
over your head with your palms flat and your elbows facing to the sides.
Inhale and press up as if you were going to push the ceiling with your
hands. Hold for 30 seconds, breathing normally. Repeat.

▸BENEFIT The palm position of this exercise isolates and strengthens the muscles
in the shoulders.

Thigh toner

Sit up straight. While drawing in your stomach muscles, curl your hands into fists and place them between your knees. Squeeze your fists with your thighs and hold for 30 seconds. Repeat.

▶**BENEFIT** Strengthens and firms those difficult-to-isolate muscles in the inner thighs.

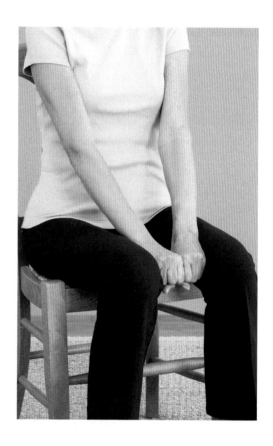

Palm clasp

Sit up straight and grab one hand with the other. Press your palms together hard for 5 seconds, then release. Do this four times. You can also do this exercise while waiting at traffic lights or watching TV.

▶**BENEFIT** This anytime-anywhere exercise strengthens the chest and arms.

▶ In the kitchen

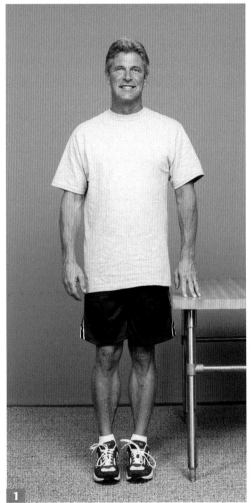 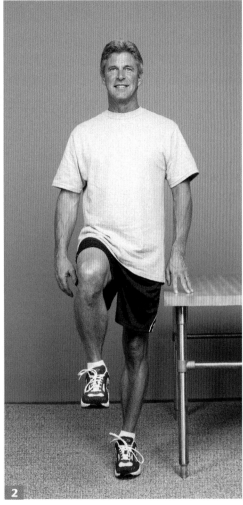

Knee raise

While waiting for water to boil, stand sideways near the kitchen counter. Place your left hand on the counter for balance. **1**

Keeping your trunk upright, transfer all your weight to your left leg and raise your right knee to hip level. **2** Hold for 5 seconds then lower your foot to the floor. Repeat with the other leg. Do five times with each leg.

▶**BENEFIT** Strengthens the thighs, hamstrings and hip extensor muscles. Working your leg muscles supports your knee, which allows it to better absorb impact while walking.

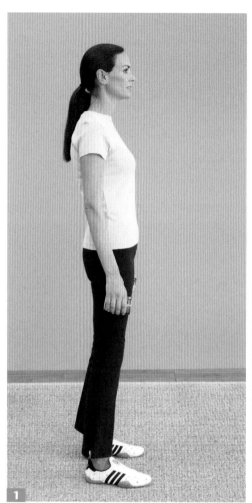 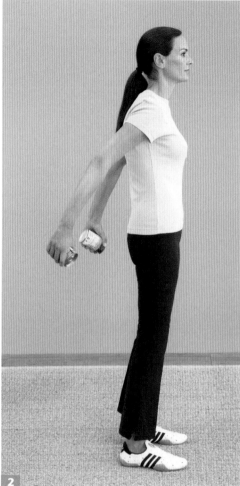

Triceps kickback

Stand with your feet hip-width apart, your back straight and your knees flexed. Grasp a full can of soup (weighing no more than 450g/1lb) in each hand and rest them against the sides of your thighs. **1**

Keeping your elbows and wrists fixed and your shoulders back, exhale and raise the cans behind you as far as is comfortable. **2** Hold for 5 seconds. Inhale and return to the starting position. Do this five times.

▶**BENEFIT** Works the triceps, which are important for pushing, such as moving a heavy shopping trolley, and lifting, such as carrying bags of groceries from the car. Tones the 'wobbly' flesh on your upper arms.

Biceps curl

Stand with your feet shoulder-width apart, holding a full can of soup in each hand by your sides, palms facing forward. **1**

Exhaling, curl your forearms toward your chest, keeping your elbows close to your sides. **2** Keep your abdominal muscles tensed and don't allow your lower back to sway. Hold for 1 second. Inhale and return to the starting position. Do this five times.

▶**BENEFIT** Works the biceps, which are important for pulling, such as yanking up weeds in the garden, and lifting, whether it's a bag of groceries or a grandchild.

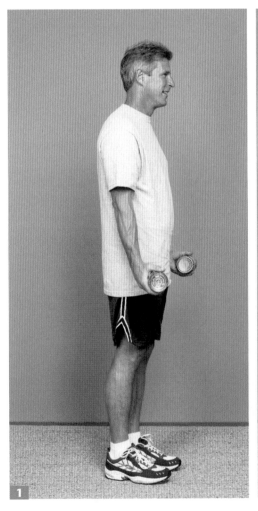

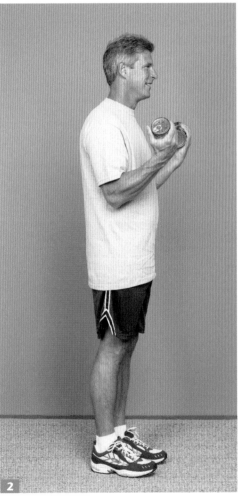

*T*his yoga-based routine stretches out the kinks and improves blood flow. It works as a morning wake-up routine, too. Do the whole routine, slowly and gently, and don't pause between movements. You will become more flexible the more you practise this.

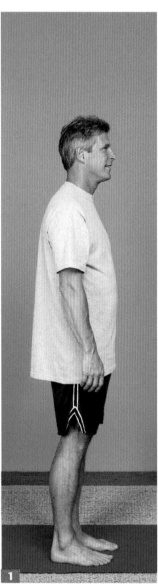 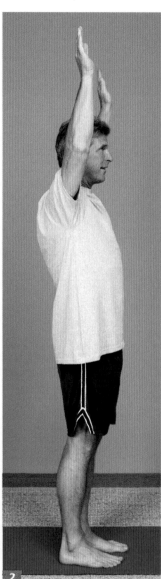 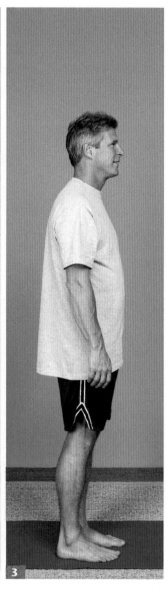

Mountain pose

Stand with your feet hip-width apart. Keep your abdominal muscles tight and don't arch your back. **1**

Inhaling, slowly raise your arms to the sides and continue until they are over your head, with your palms facing forward. **2**

Exhaling, slowly lower your arms. **3** Repeat.

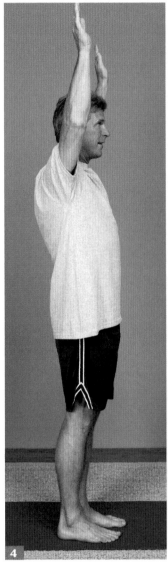
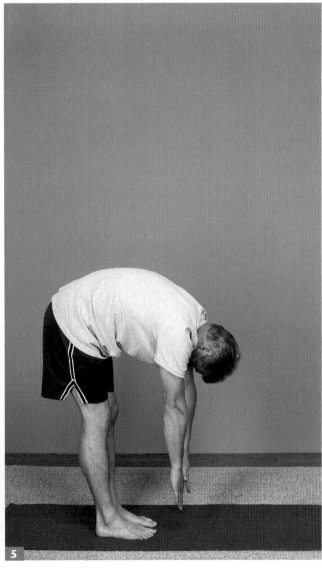

Standing forward bend

Inhale and repeat the mountain pose so that your arms are extended above your head, palms facing forward. **4**

Exhaling, tuck in your bottom and bend forward at the waist, keeping a slight bend in your elbows and knees. **5** Try to touch the floor or your ankles or shins, depending on what is comfortable. Roll back up to the starting position. Repeat.

▶ **CAUTION** If you have back pain, place a small stool or a stack of books about 30cm (12in) high by your feet and reach towards that.

STEP 5 Sensitize with exercise   163

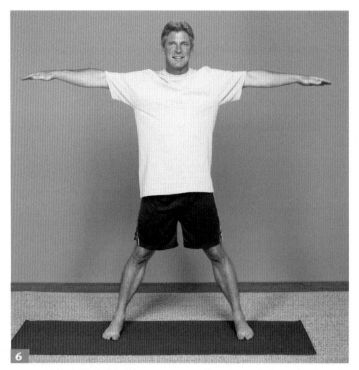

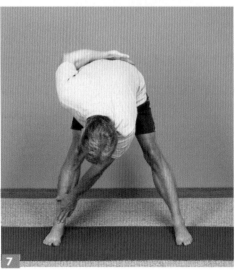

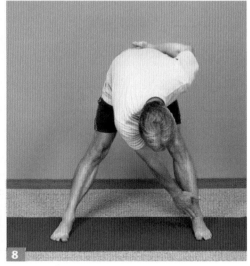

Triangle pose

Stand with your feet 60-90cm (2-3ft) apart – wider than hip-width – with your toes facing forward.

Inhaling, raise your arms to the sides until they reach shoulder level, palms down, so your upper body forms a T.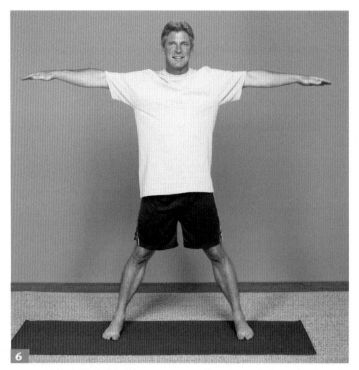

Exhaling, bend forward at the waist and reach with your left hand towards your right ankle, foot or calf (whichever feels most comfortable), placing your right hand on the small of your back. 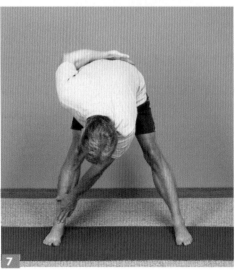 Return to the T position and repeat on the other side. 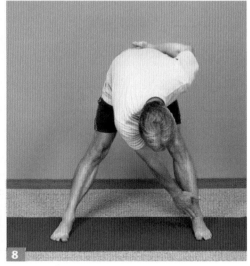 Do this three times.

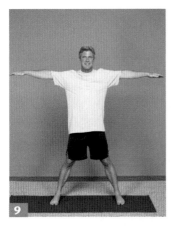

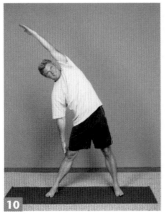

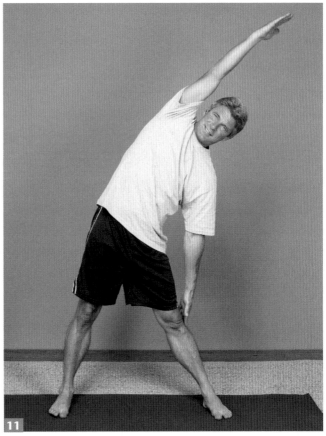

Standing side stretch

Stand with your feet 60-90cm (2-3ft) apart – wider than hip-width – and raise your arms to the sides to form a T. **9**

Exhaling, bend to the right and grasp your right leg with your right hand just below the knee, while bending your left arm slightly over your head so your left elbow moves closer to your ear. **10**

Inhaling, return to the starting position and repeat on the other side. **11** Do this three times.

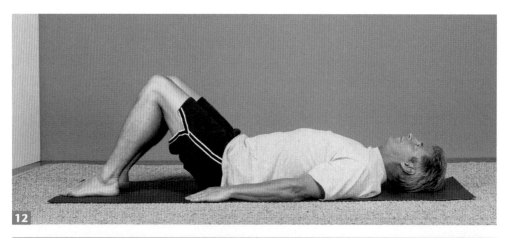

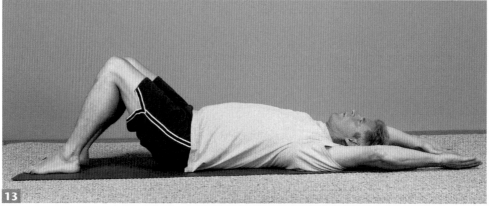

Touchdown tilt

Lie on your back with your knees bent and about hip-width apart, with your arms at your sides and your hands on the floor, palms down. **12**

Inhaling, raise your hands over your head. **13** Let your back arch slightly and touch your hands on the floor above your head or, if it's more comfortable, rest them by your ears with your elbows bent.

Exhaling, bring your arms back to your sides and flatten your back gently towards the floor. Do this three times.

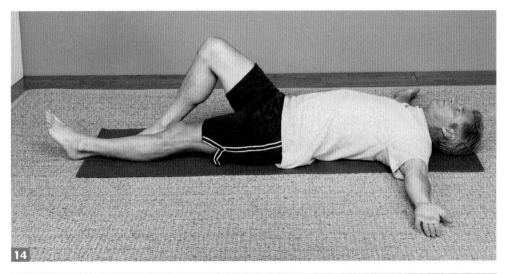

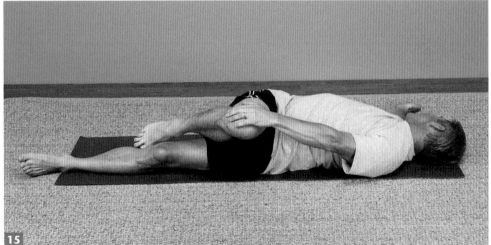

Lying twist

Lie on your back with your right knee bent so that your foot is on the floor near your left knee.

Exhaling, turn your head to the right and use your left hand to gently pull your right knee towards the floor on the left.

Inhale and return to the starting position. Repeat on the other side. Do this three times.

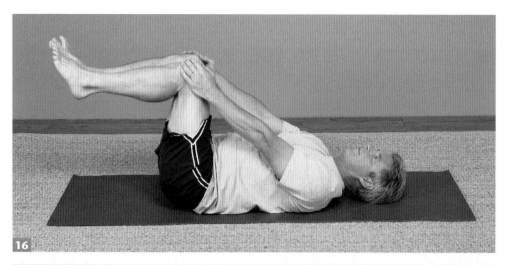

16

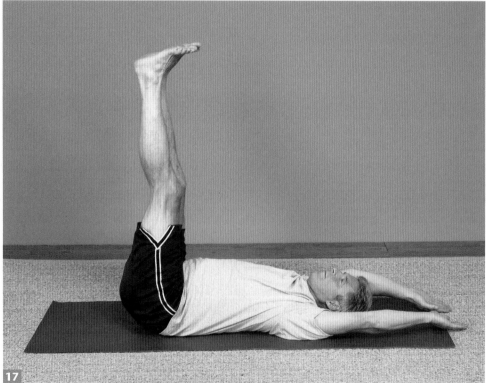

17

Upward raised legs

Lie on your back and use your hands to pull your knees towards your chest, keeping them slightly apart. 16

Inhaling, extend your legs straight up from your hips so the bottoms of your feet point towards the ceiling. At the same time, extend your arms above your head to touch the floor, keeping your chin tucked into your chest. (Place a small pillow under your head if it's more comfortable.) 17

Exhaling, return to the starting position. Do this three times.

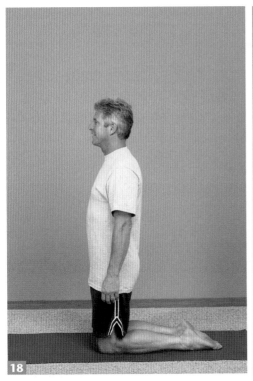

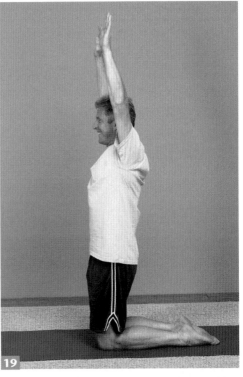

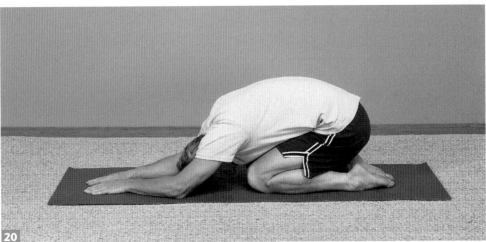

Relaxation pose

Kneel on a rug or mat with your knees slightly apart and your arms at your sides. 18

Inhaling, raise your arms straight over your head. (If that feels uncomfortable, raise your arms in front of you at a 45-degree angle.) 19

Exhaling, bend forward at the waist and lower your extended hands and forearms to the floor, moving your hips back so that you are sitting on your feet. 20 Hold for 30 to 60 seconds. Do this exercise once only.

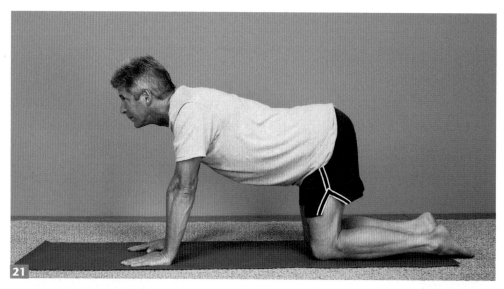

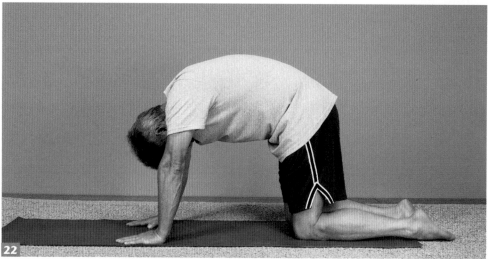

Cat pose

From the relaxation pose, get on your hands and knees. Inhaling and keeping your weight distributed evenly on your arms and legs, raise your chin and arch your back so it makes a gentle U-shaped dip towards the floor. Move at your pelvis, sticking your bottom out. **21**

Exhaling, lower your head, tuck in your bottom and tilt your pelvis to round your spine, starting with your lower back and progressing through your middle and upper back. **22** At the end of the pose your head should be slightly lower than your hips. Do this three times.

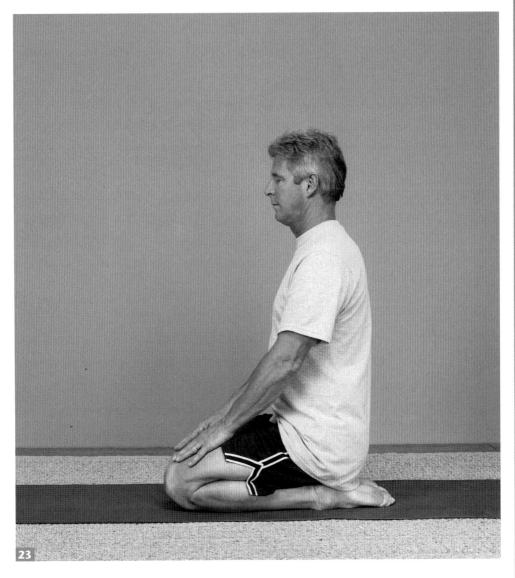

Kneeling rest pose

From the cat pose, lower your hips until you are in a kneeling position. Keeping your back straight, rest your hands lightly on your thighs. **23** Close your eyes and breathe slowly for 1 minute.

If this position is uncomfortable for you, try placing a pillow between your feet and your buttocks.

STEP 6 Master your moods

Calm down. Relax. Take it easy. That's what we want you to do next. Counteracting the stresses, strains and irritations of daily life can enable your body to handle blood sugar more effectively and even help you to store less abdominal fat. In addition lowering your body's levels of so-called stress hormones will even make you less hungry.

Dedicated relaxation is part of the 10 Per Cent Plan. In fact, we want you to set aside 20 minutes a day in which to purposefully unwind.

From deep breathing drills to exercises using your imagination, this chapter suggests plenty of ways to spend those 20 minutes. You should also treat yourself to an occasional massage and make sure that you get enough sleep, both of which can help to lower your blood sugar levels. All of these approaches will help you to stick to your goals and focus on a truly important aspect of your life: your health.

Good reasons to relax

Eating healthily and taking exercise every day are pillars of any programme for managing diabetes or losing weight. The 10 Per Cent Plan brings in a third element that may be almost as important: managing stress.

Research is now beginning to reveal just how important stress management is when it comes to diabetes. One study, at Duke University in Durham, North Carolina, found that when people used easy relaxation techniques such as the ones you will learn here, their A1C numbers (an indication of blood sugar levels over several months) dropped significantly. In fact, after a year about one-third of the volunteers had lowered their A1C levels by as much as if they'd taken diabetes drugs.

Track your sugar trends

Studies find that stress affects blood sugar differently from one person to the next. How do your sugar levels change when you are all charged up? To find out, each time you check your blood glucose level, rate how stressed you feel at that moment on a scale of 1 to 10, with 1 being a sunny day at the beach and 10 being the worst day of your life. Write down the number next to your reading. After two weeks, look at the numbers together (it may help to plot them on a graph) to see how much your blood sugar swings in response to various levels of stress.

And those results were in addition to the benefits they gained through diet and exercise. So why does taming tension bring down blood sugar?

STRESS HORMONES RAISE BLOOD SUGAR When you're on edge, your body pumps out stress hormones, such as cortisol, to help you to react to danger (part of the 'fight or flight' response). These hormones speed up your heartbeat and breathing and also send glucose stores into the blood to make energy immediately available to your muscles. The result: higher blood sugar.

STRESS CONTRIBUTES TO INSULIN RESISTANCE Stress hormones make it more difficult for the pancreas to secrete the insulin needed to remove glucose from the blood. Some stress hormones may also contribute to insulin resistance.

STRESS LEADS TO WEIGHT GAIN A major reason to keep chronic stress in check is that cortisol is known to increase appetite. Stress makes you eat more. It also encourages cells in your abdomen to conserve fat. In other words, it packs on the pounds around your belly, which are precisely the ones that seriously increase your risk of a heart attack.

Regularly practising our relaxation methods will help to lower your levels of stress hormones to reverse this trend. It should also help you to stick to your eating and exercise goals. Think about it: when you're stressed, you are probably tempted to eat whatever fatty, high-calorie snacks are within reach. You are also less likely to think about going out for a nice long walk when you're busy fretting over deadlines, family problems or that fight with your partner. When you practise the art of relaxation, you'll step back and see the big picture, and your true priorities – including taking care of your body – will emerge.

Mastering stress levels has other beneficial side effects. Specifically, it helps to ward off emotional problems that are linked with poor blood sugar control, particularly depression and anger. (Exercise has similar effects, which is another reason why it is important to follow Step Five.)

Since stress exists in both your mind and body, our stress-relieving techniques tackle it on both fronts. Progress in one automatically creates gains in the other, so if you try two or three of these techniques, you will reap real results.

Diabetes UK endorses the use of relaxation exercises to help reduce blood glucose levels, but recommends consulting your doctor beforehand.

1 Learn to breathe well

ACTION You probably think that breathing comes naturally, but the way we instinctively breathed as babies is not the way most of us do it as stressed-out adults. The reason for this is that tension causes the entire body to tighten up. That makes your breathing shallow and fast, with less air going into the bases of your lungs. It may sound trivial, but it's not. When your body has trouble getting enough oxygen, it feels even more stressed, which can lead to a faster heartbeat, higher blood pressure and increased levels of stress hormones that raise blood sugar.

Remarkably, simply breathing more evenly, slowly and deeply can turn off the body's stress switch and bring down blood sugar. In fact, there is no better way to instantly de-stress. The trick is to make your lungs expand as much as possible, filling them with air from the bottom up. To do that, you need to breathe with your belly and stretch your diaphragm muscle between your chest and abdominal cavity, at the base of your lungs. If you're accustomed to shallow breathing, this may feel unnatural at first, and you may even need to strengthen your diaphragm to do it correctly. The following exercises will develop that muscle and remind your body how to breathe the way nature intended.

SIGH STRATEGICALLY

Do you ever find yourself sighing and yawning when under stress? That's your body's way of getting you to breathe more

A workout for your chest

If you're accustomed to taking short, shallow breaths, your chest and diaphragm muscles are probably out of shape. Here's how to get them fit.

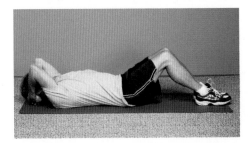 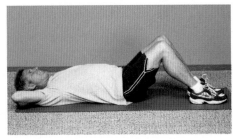

To help your chest expand and boost lung capacity, lie on the floor with your knees bent and your feet flat on the floor. Place your hands behind your head and bring your elbows together so they are nearly touching. As you inhale, slowly let your elbows drop to the sides so your arms are flat on the floor when your lungs are full. As you exhale, raise your elbows again.

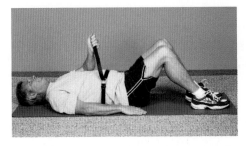 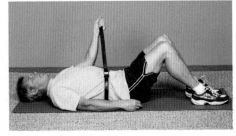

Strengthen your diaphragm by giving the muscle some resistance while you are breathing. Wrap a belt around your abdomen, then lie on the floor with your knees bent and your feet flat on the floor. As you exhale, pull on the belt to put pressure on your abdomen. As you inhale, slowly let up on the pressure, but keep the belt tight enough so that your diaphragm has to push against it to fill your lungs. An alternative is to press on your abdomen with your hands.

deeply. Start your stress-reduction programme by building on that sighing instinct. Intentional sighing will help to dissolve physical tension and get more oxygen into your system.

1. While sitting or standing straight, with your hands at your sides or resting on your knees, let the air rush out of your lungs as if you were deeply relieved that a stressful event has passed (even if it hasn't).

2. For the moment, forget about how you are breathing in. Just take another breath naturally and let it rush out again.

3. Repeat 10 times for a total of 12 sighs. By the time you have finished, it won't feel as if you're sighing any more. Instead, you will be breathing deeply.

PRACTISE ABDOMINAL BREATHING

Another way to make sure that you are breathing properly – that is from your belly, not your chest – is to practise this deep-breathing exercise. Deep breathing makes tense muscles relax indirectly by signalling to your brain that you have entered a state of rest and peace. Do this exercise daily or any time you notice that stress is getting the better of you.

1. Find a quiet place and sit comfortably with your back flat against the back of a chair. Place one hand on your chest and the other on your stomach, then breathe normally. Pay attention to which hand moves the most as you inhale and exhale. If it's the hand on your chest, the lower areas of your lungs are not filling with air.

2. Take a deep breath through your nose. Inhale slowly so you can't hear your breathing; if the rush of air makes a noise, you are inhaling too quickly. Fill the bottom sections of your lungs first so your diaphragm pushes the hand on your stomach outwards. Continue to inhale until you fill the upper parts of your lungs, making the hand on your chest rise slightly.

3. Hold your breath for a moment and think of the word *relax*.

4. Exhale slowly and naturally without forcing the air out (it's fine if you can hear the air escaping). Continue breathing in and out slowly for several minutes.

Quiz
How best to deal with stress

You have plenty of options for managing stress. Do you need them all? Knowing more about what bothers you can help you to find the right techniques to combat your stress. Circle any statement that is true of you.

◆ I find it hard to concentrate on the things I need to do.

■ I often find it difficult to get going in the morning.

● If another driver cuts in ahead of me in traffic, I move up close behind him.

◆ It's common for me to find myself thinking about work problems at home.

● I get very impatient in slow-moving queues at the supermarket or bank.

◆ I often feel tense.

■ I really don't feel I have a lot to look forward to.

● Most people will lie or stab others in the back to get ahead.

◆ My mind is plagued by unsettling thoughts.

● When people are rude or irritating to me, I give them a piece of my mind.

■ When I need to make a decision, it's hard for me to work out what to do.

◆ I worry quite a lot.

■ I don't feel like talking to people as much as I used to.

◆ It's hard for me to unwind and relax.

● When I feel someone is wrong, there's likely to be an argument.

● People who talk about how difficult their life is are simply trying to get attention.

◆ I've experienced sexual difficulties recently.

■ I'm so sick of myself, dying would seem like an escape.

◆ I feel insecure much of the time.

● When I'm around someone I dislike, I don't care if I seem rude.

● Most people can't really be trusted.

■ Activities that used to be fun don't seem that way any more.

● People who tell me what to do usually don't know what they're talking about.

◆ I've been arguing more with my spouse/partner lately.

■ I often feel lonely.

● I've been known to throw things or hit people when I get really angry.

■ There are a lot of days when I can't seem to shake off sad feelings.

■ I feel tired and lethargic a lot of the time.

◆ I find it difficult to get a good night's sleep lately.

Continue overleaf

Quiz (continued)

- If someone pays me a compliment, I wonder what they want from me.

- It's not unusual for me to break down and cry three or more times a week.

- I often have aches and pains even if I haven't been exercising.

- My life has been nothing but a series of failures.

- I'm not sure I can handle everything I need to do.

- I don't really enjoy being around people very much.

- Most people would break the law more often if they knew they wouldn't get caught.

What your score means

Count how many of each type of statement you circled.

____ ◆ diamond
____ ■ square
____ ● circle

If you circled four or more ◆ statements, stress is a problem for you. Start by doing deep breathing and correcting irrational thinking, which will produce results fast. When your schedule allows, take time to do progressive muscle relaxation (see page 179), autogenics (see page 180) and imagery (see page 183).

If you circled four or more ■ statements, it's likely that you are depressed. Correcting irrational thinking is likely to benefit you most. If you continue to feel low for more than two weeks, however, seek help from a professional therapist.

If you circled four or more ● statements, your biggest problem is anger. You will benefit most from deep breathing, correcting irrational thinking and following our tips for curbing anger.

2 Dissolve muscle tension

ACTION Whereas deep breathing works by sending a signal to your brain that you are relaxing, the following exercises work by tackling muscle tension head-on. The first approach we want you to try is progressive muscle relaxation. Studies have found that regularly practising this technique can lower blood sugar enough to significantly reduce the risk of complications such as kidney disease and eye damage. It can also bring down high blood pressure and help to guard against heart disease.

The idea behind progressive muscle relaxation sounds like a contradiction: to make muscles relax, you must first make them tense. The reason it works is that we don't usually notice a lot of the tension in our muscles. Tightening them draws attention to it so you can focus on letting it drain away.

DO A 20-MINUTE **TENSION TAMER**

Twenty minutes is all the time you need in order to do a full progressive relaxation routine. To gain the maximum benefit, try to practise this at least once a day, perhaps at bedtime.

Help!

Whenever I'm stressed or upset I reach for food.

It's no surprise that food is tied to feelings. As children, our parents nurtured and rewarded us with food. As adults, we equate food with socializing, relaxing and having fun. As a result, eating food can be comforting when you're feeling low or stressed, and stimulating when you're feeling bored.

- First, make sure that you are not genuinely hungry. If it is more than 4 or 5 hours since you last ate, have a low-fat snack, such as a piece of fruit. Note what you feel like eating. If any food would satisfy you, you are probably truly hungry. If you crave a specific food, your 'hunger' is probably driven by emotions.
- Wait it out. Cravings often vanish as fast as they appear. Instead of eating, play with your dog, call a friend or do a small chore.
- Get out of the house, or at least the kitchen. In other words, take yourself out of the way of temptation.
- Take a detour after work to defuse stress so that you're not tempted to raid your fridge and larder when you get home. A stroll through the park should do the trick.
- Find other ways to indulge. Food isn't the only way to treat yourself. You may find that you can raise your spirits by shopping, reading a novel or having a massage.

1. While either lying down or sitting in a comfortable chair that supports your head, close your eyes and start by mentally scanning your body for places that feel tense.

2. Follow the serenity sequence on the opposite page, clenching each muscle area as tightly as you can and holding for 5 seconds. Take about 20 seconds to gradually release the tension, consciously relaxing your muscles as much as possible, then move on to the next area.

3. Silently repeat a soothing thought, such as 'I am totally calm' or 'Goodbye, tension'.

RELAX TO A EURYTHMIC BEAT

Eurythmics is a music education technique developed by a Swiss composer who believed the body is finely tuned to musical rhythms. Some relaxation therapists have adopted his methods to combine full-body muscle relaxation with deep breathing in a meditative rhythm set to the tick-tock of a metronome. Here's how to do it.

• Set a metronome so that it ticks off one beat per second (or use a ticking clock).

• Inhale for a count of six, hold your breath for one count, then exhale for a count of six. (You can take more than six beats to inhale and exhale if your lungs take longer than that to fill.)

• Repeat the breathing exercise, but this time, gradually tense all your muscles for the count of six. Hold the tension for one count, relax your body for a count of six, and pause for a count of one.

• Continue tensing and relaxing your entire body in time with your breathing, or use each cycle of counting to focus on specific areas, such as your arms, legs, torso and head.

ARM YOURSELF WITH AUTOGENICS

Like progressive muscle relaxation, autogenics (a form of self-hypnosis) harnesses the power of the imagination to make the body relax. Therapists sometimes use it in conjunction with biofeedback (a process that uses machines to monitor body

Calves and feet Curl your toes towards the floor, keeping your heels flat, then relax.

Shins Raise your toes off the floor, then relax.

Thighs Push your heels against the floor, then relax.

Buttocks Squeeze your buttocks together, then relax.

Abdomen Pull your navel in towards your backbone, then relax.

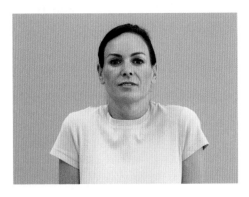

Hands Clench your fists, then relax.

Arms Bend your dominant arm at the elbow and tense your biceps and lower arm as hard as you can without clenching your fist. Relax and repeat with the other arm.

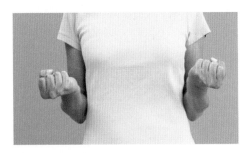

Shoulders Shrug your shoulders up towards your ears as far as is comfortable. As you release, note the relaxation you feel in your neck.

Neck Press your head into the back of your chair, then relax. Bend your neck and move your chin down onto your chest. As you relax, let your head return to a comfortable upright position.

Jaw Tighten your jaw so your back teeth clench together. Gradually relax, ending with your lips slightly parted.

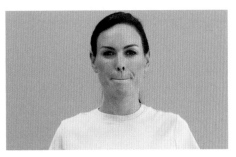

Lips Press your lips and front teeth together, then relax.

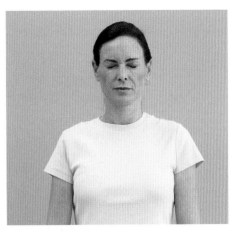

Eyes Squeeze your eyes shut as tightly as you can, then relax, keeping your eyelids closed.

Forehead Raise your eyebrows and wrinkle your forehead as tightly as you can, then relax while picturing your forehead becoming smooth. Next, deeply furrow your brow into a frown and relax.

functions such as sweating or brain activity in order to help manage stress-related conditions), but you don't need to be hooked to a machine to benefit from it. All you need is a quiet room and a comfortable chair that supports your head, back and arms. Or you can sit slightly stooped on a stool, with your arms resting on your thighs and your hands hanging loosely between your knees.

Once you are settled into position with your eyes closed, do the following sequence.

1. Concentrate your attention on your dominant arm, usually the right. Slowly repeat 'My right arm is heavy' in your mind and imagine the arm actually becoming heavier. Pause after the statement, repeating it four times.

2. Do the same with your left arm.

3. Next, repeat the exercise using the words 'Both my arms are heavy'.

4. Concentrate on your right leg and slowly repeat 'My right leg is heavy' four times.

5. Do the same with your left leg, then both legs.

6. Repeat the exercise, but this time use the word *warm* instead of *heavy* and imagine your limbs becoming warmer.

Once you are familiar with this technique, you can do another exercise in which you imagine your limbs becoming heavier and warmer at the same time. It's possible that you will enter a trance-like state, which is fine. When you have finished the exercise, simply mark its completion by telling yourself, 'When I open my eyes, I will be refreshed and alert.'

SCHEDULE A **MASSAGE**

Who could imagine that something as luxuriously indulgent as a massage could actually help you to manage diabetes? But it can. Anecdotal evidence suggests that a massage can temporarily lower blood sugar by between 1.1mmol/l and 3.9mmol/l, or even more. Massage helps you relax, lowering levels of stress hormones, which in turn lowers blood glucose. Massage also boosts blood circulation, which is often less than perfect in people with diabetes. In short, massage is not just about being pampered; it's also about your health.

Of course, a massage from a professional massage therapist is best. Check local gyms and alternative therapy centres to find massage services, or ask your doctor for a referral. Swedish massage, the most common type, is the one generally used for relaxation. Because your blood sugar could drop during the massage, tell the therapist that you have diabetes, and be prepared with a sugary snack. If you take insulin, be aware that massage may increase your body's uptake of the insulin at the injection site and send your blood sugar down rapidly.

If you can't afford to pay for a professional massage or don't want to spend the money, ask a friend or relative to give you a massage using light, unscented lotion or massage oil. You can also give yourself a soothing mini-massage. In one small study at New Mexico State University, the blood-sugar levels in patients with Type 2 diabetes fell after six weekly stress-relieving sessions that included gripping the fingers, squeezing the arms and pressing the head. The following massages are easy to carry out on yourself.

- Grasp and twist your right forefinger between the thumb and fingers of your left hand, sliding from the base to the tip of the finger as you twist. Repeat twice with each finger of your right hand, then repeat on your left hand.

- Take hold of your right forearm so that your left thumb is positioned just below your right palm. Use your thumb to stroke up the forearm to the elbow. Turn your arm over and massage the top of the forearm as well, then repeat on the other arm.

- Place four fingertips of each hand on top of your head and press down, moving your fingertips in a circular motion.

3 Picture serenity now

ACTION

Tranquil thoughts are like water bubbling from a spring that percolates into a flowing stream and nourishes the world around it. Stressful thoughts, on the other hand, are like an overwhelming flood. Control the water, and you keep havoc under control so that everything remains calm, serene and marked by the pure, quiet sound of gurgling.

In case you didn't notice, all that talk about tranquil, flowing water makes use of imagery, a powerful technique for focusing thoughts on peaceful mental pictures and triggering the feelings that go with them. You may be sceptical about such techniques. But it is clear that even subtle thoughts and feelings can have an impact on blood sugar. For example, laboratory mice bred to have diabetes have higher blood sugar when they are conditioned to merely *anticipate* a minor annoyance such as the floor under their feet moving.

The following exercises use a variety of meditative techniques that harness some form of imagery. To do them, find a quiet place where you can sit undisturbed for up to 20 minutes. Use the deep-breathing techniques that you have already learned while you take your mind through the exercises. To make the images easier to conjure up, consider recording the instructions on an audiotape so you don't have to memorize or refer to them.

Don't worry if you find unwanted thoughts intruding while you're using imagery. When thoughts shoved into the recesses of your mind start to move into your consciousness, it's a sign that you're letting go of the stress that was holding them back. Simply allow them to move through your mind, then return to the exercise.

COLOUR YOUR WORLD

There is no need to conjure up detailed scenes to begin with. Many people find that even picturing colours can promote feelings of peace and calm.

1. Close your eyes and imagine your entire field of vision filled with a single colour. It doesn't matter which colour you choose; try different ones and settle on whatever colour is easiest to hold in your mind.

2. Imagine the colour becoming punctuated with areas of lighter and darker shades. Picture the shades slowly drifting about like clouds in the sky.

3. Next, imagine another colour appearing in a simple geometric shape, such as a circle or triangle. Focus on this new colour while you take several deep breaths, then imagine that another colour appears in a different shape.

4. Allow the shapes to start moving around slowly in your mind's eye and give them different dimensions, so a square

becomes a cube or a triangle becomes a cone. Let them slowly tumble and move through space. Add other shapes if you wish, or change the colour of the background.

TAKE A MENTAL GETAWAY

Now it's time to really let your imagination loose. Even though you can't escape to a beautiful, peaceful place whenever stress rears its ugly head, if you can imagine such a place – including all the sights, sounds, smells and even the temperature – you can experience it. The scenario you choose is up to you. Here is one example.

1. Picture yourself on a mountaintop surrounded by lush tropical vegetation but open to the sky, so you are bathed in sunlight. Note the deep blue colour of the sky, feel the sun's rays soothing your body, smell the fragrance of the flowers all around, and hear the patter of drops falling off leaves after a recent rain. Look far below and see a tranquil beach on the shore of a placid lake.

2. Take yourself to the shore of the lake and imagine walking along the soft sand. You are completely alone, but you find a boat tied to a dock. After untying the mooring rope, lie down on soft blankets inside the boat and watch the clouds as you drift on the calm water. The boat rocks gently, and waves gurgle under the hull as you drink in the warmth and feel the soft movement of a breeze. You feel a deep sense of relaxation as you drift between the water and the clouds.

TRY THE 'PINK BUBBLE' TECHNIQUE

Build on your powers of imagination to create more sophisticated images that are tied to your goals or desires. Use this very simple but potentially powerful technique when everyday stresses – an irritable boss, family difficulties, an illness – seem to prevent you from realizing your dreams, which can create a sense of powerlessness and frustration.

1. Sit quietly with your eyes closed and imagine that a dream or goal has already been fulfilled – perhaps you have found a new job, you are on your ideal holiday, or you are retired and living somewhere warm and beautiful.

2. Imagine the scene becoming surrounded by a translucent pink bubble, a colour associated with the heart. Watch as the scene enclosed in the pink bubble begins to lift and slowly float away. Breathe deeply as you imagine the scene floating through the universe, gathering energy for a time when it will return to you. Let go of frustration as you wait for the day the scene comes back.

ACTION 4 Use real-life anti-stress strategies

Fights with spouses, health problems, money worries. Things happen. To everyone, not just you. When they do, how do you react? Do you panic and imagine that divorce, death or financial ruin is imminent? You see, it's not necessarily the things that life throws at you that cause stress (and raise blood sugar levels), but rather your reaction to them.

Two common types of thinking can act against you. One is assuming the worst – for example, believing that because your boss is in a bad mood you are going to be fired. The other is believing that you, other people and the world in general have to live up to certain standards – which leads to frustration and disappointment when they inevitably don't. Stress-inducing thoughts often stem from irrational beliefs such as:

- It's necessary that everyone likes me.
- If people disapprove of me, I must be wrong or bad.
- I have to be competent in everything I do.
- My value as a person depends on what I achieve.
- It's terrible when things aren't the way I want.
- People are the victims of their circumstances.
- I'm entitled to a good life and should never experience pain.

By identifying such underlying beliefs you will find it easier to counter this negative thinking that can cause additional stress and bring you down.

According to a recent joint report by Diabetes UK in Northern Ireland and Action for Mental Health, between 20 and 30 per cent of people with diabetes experience depression – a rate approximately three times higher than in the general population. The report also found that depression is directly related to poor self-care in people with diabetes.

STOP NEGATIVE THOUGHTS

To stop negative reactions in their tracks, try the following strategies.

1. Start by writing down (or thinking clearly about) exactly what happened in an upsetting situation. Take a just-the-facts approach and skip any value judgments or conjectures. Examples of facts might be: your boss seemed irritated this morning; your child disobeyed you; your spouse worked late.

2. Note what you are telling yourself about this supposedly terrible event and how it makes you feel. Be sure to include all your assumptions, predictions and beliefs. If your boss is irritated, these might include: 'I must have done something wrong'; 'He's always in a bad mood when I'm around, so he must hate me'; or 'He acted like this the last time he let someone go, so he's probably going to again.'

3. Challenge your assumptions. Is your boss's irritation really about you, or could there be another cause? Is he really this way all the time? Hasn't he been angry many times without firing anybody?

4. Change what you tell yourself to fit the evidence. For example, 'My boss is irritated, but he's always that way. It probably has nothing to do with me'; or 'I can't be responsible for my boss's mood – only for my own.'

A question of perspective

Whenever you feel stressed by the way someone treats you or when a difficult situation arises, keep the following in mind.

- **Stress is about me, not the situation** An aeroplane flight may panic someone who has never flown but seem mind-numbingly dull to a business traveller. The right perspective will enable you to handle any situation.
- **What's done is done** Lots of things happen for reasons that are beyond your control, and thinking 'would have', 'could have' or 'should have' won't help you to deal with an existing situation. Instead, think in future-oriented terms, such as 'I hope' or 'next time'.
- **Nobody's perfect, including me** Expect a reasonable amount of disappointment and failure from both yourself and other people, then adopt an attitude of forgiveness.

PUT A **STOP SIGN** IN YOUR BRAIN

In research conducted at Duke University, one technique that proved helpful for people with diabetes was a simple method known as thought stopping. Use it whenever negative or irrational thinking starts to get the better of you.

1. Close your eyes and imagine a situation in which the stressful thought might enter your head. Set a timer for 3 minutes and continue contemplating the stressful thought.

2. When the timer goes off, shout 'Stop!' If you wish, punctuate your exclamation with a physical sign, such as standing up or clapping your hands. (This may seem awkward at first, but the forcefulness of the statement is part of what makes it work. As you become more experienced with the technique, you can say the word more quietly or think it to yourself.) Try to keep your mind blank for 30 seconds, and if the thought comes back, shout 'Stop!' again.

3. Replace the distressing thought with a more positive, rational thought. For example, if the stressful thought is 'I can't do this; I'm worthless', instead say to yourself, 'There are many valuable things I can do.'

LEARN TO HANDLE HOSTILITY

Do you always feel at war with the people around you? Do you lean on the horn if the person in front of you is driving too slowly? Is your first response to a difficult situation to get angry? If so, you may have the type of personality that has been shown to raise blood glucose levels.

Researchers have long suspected that anger and hostility play a role in heart disease. More recent findings suggest that people who are typically angry or show related traits such as cynicism, rage and aggression also tend to have higher blood sugar and insulin resistance. Angry or hostile people are also more likely to overeat. One study, for example, found that people who tended to be hostile consumed 600 more kcal a day than people who were less angry.

You can't change your personality, but you can modify your angry thinking and behaviour. Start by using deep breathing and the other techniques you've just learned. Programmes using stress management and relaxation training to manage anger have been shown to lower rates of heart attack, and researchers at Duke University believe the same approaches can help to control blood sugar. Take these practical steps to prevent momentary flare-ups from getting out of hand.

GET AWAY Sometimes the only way to keep from blowing your top is to leave the situation that is provoking you until you can calm down. The best bet is to take an

Negative thoughts workshop

Catching yourself in the act of negative thinking is the first step towards stopping it. When you notice you have a negative thought, write it down in the left column. Then find a way to 'spin' the thought into a more positive one. (We have given you a few examples to get you started.) To gain more mileage from this exercise, speak the positive thoughts into a tape recorder and play the messages back to yourself.

NEGATIVE THOUGHT	POSITIVE THOUGHT
I'm disorganized and can't get everything done.	If I take more time for myself, I'll have more energy and focus.
I'll never reach my weight-loss goal.	If I can lose just 500g (1lb), that's a good start.

exercise break. If it is not possible to remove yourself physically from the situation, distract your mind by counting up to 10. It's a simple technique but it works.

BE SPECIFIC When confronting someone you are angry with, don't launch into a long list of perceived faults and slights. Instead, focus on the one thing that is really bothering you – and be sure to work out what that is before you speak up. Say exactly what you would like to see changed to make the situation better.

AVOID INSULTS It may be tempting to 'explain' how another person is being inconsiderate or boorish, but you won't make headway in solving the real issue (getting more help from a spouse, how much money to spend on holiday) if the other person is too busy being defensive to listen.

You will also help yourself by seeking out the company of positive people and limiting your exposure to negative or irritating people.

5 ACTION Lower blood sugar with sleep

A really basic way to feel less stressed during the day – and one that many of us fail to capitalize on – is to get enough sleep at night.

Wouldn't it be great if you could go to bed and wake up with better blood sugar control? In effect, that may be what you do when you get adequate sleep. Recent research suggests that not getting the sleep you need may contribute to insulin resistance. One reason is that poor sleepers often experience sleep apnoea, a condition that interferes with normal breathing and has been linked to diabetes. But there is also evidence that sleep by itself helps the body to use glucose more efficiently.

One study found that people who had only about 5 hours of sleep had 40 per cent lower insulin sensitivity than people who had about 8 hours. Are you getting enough sleep? Probably not. Some 20 million British adults suffer from sleep problems at some stage in their lives, while half of Britons say they are sleep deprived. More than one-third of us are sleeping six hours or less each night – losing a month's sleep every year.

If this sounds like a problem with a simple (and enjoyable) solution, it is. Spend more time in bed. But getting enough sleep is as much about quality as quantity, and it's not always easy to drift off when you want to, especially when you are under stress. Fortunately, if you have followed the 10 Per Cent Plan up to this point, you are already doing plenty that will help you to achieve the right amount of good quality sleep: eating healthily, exercising and managing stress. If you still need help, however, try the following tips.

DON'T SLEEP IN Lying in at weekends seems an obvious way to catch up on your sleep, but it may be doing more harm than good by throwing your body out of rhythm, which can make it more difficult to get to sleep at night. If you want to add sleep time, go to bed earlier and get up at the usual time. Then try to stick to your new schedule so that your body clock knows when to cue feelings of sleepiness at night.

RESERVE YOUR BEDROOM FOR SLEEP Keep the TV out of the bedroom, and don't pay bills or do other paperwork in bed.

SUPPRESS YOUR MENTAL ENERGY AT NIGHT Put down a gripping book well ahead of bedtime, and if at all possible, don't start conversations that could lead to disagreements.

LEAVE YOUR WORRIES ON PAPER If you are bombarded by worries at night, take half an hour before bed to record your concerns and jot down possible solutions. When you feel you have dealt with an issue, you are more likely to drift off.

IF YOU CAN'T GET TO SLEEP, STOP TRYING If you can't sleep after 30 minutes, get out of bed, or you will only become frustrated with your efforts to fall asleep. (In one US study, volunteers who were offered a financial incentive to fall asleep quickly took longer to nod off than those who were not under any pressure.) Keep the lights low and pick up a boring book or tune into a dull TV programme until you feel sleepy again.

IF YOU WAKE UP DURING THE NIGHT, STAY IN BED You will have a better chance of falling asleep again, and your body will be getting rest even if you are not sleeping.

diab

etes

(di•a•be•tes), *noun*

1. A metabolic disorder usually
characterized by inadequate
secretion or utilization of insulin
and excessive amounts of glucose
in the blood and urine.

2. A condition causing high blood
sugar, which can be lowered
using massage, herbs and other
alternative approaches, as well
as with lifestyle changes and
medications.

PART THREE

Beyond the 10 Per Cent Plan

Other
natural
approaches

Well-timed eating, balanced meals, healthy portion sizes, exercise, stress relief: these are the essential natural solutions to diabetes contained in the 10 Per Cent Plan. Are there other measures beyond these that can help to keep blood sugar under control? Yes.

In this chapter, you will read about the most promising alternative approaches to managing diabetes and its complications.

These approaches, from acupuncture and herbs to minerals and magnet therapy, are not officially part of the plan because their effects are less well studied than those of diet and exercise. Certainly, none of them can *replace* diet and exercise if you want to lose weight and improve your health long-term, but some of them may help. Weigh the evidence for yourself and decide, after consulting your doctor, whether you want to try any of them.

Modern medicine has given us an array of weapons to fight diabetes, many of which weren't available even a decade ago. Take the best-selling drug metformin (Glucophage). It dams the release of glucose from the liver, slows the absorption of glucose from food, lowers blood levels of triglycerides (which helps to fight heart disease), and may even help people with diabetes to lose weight. But don't give chemists and synthetic compounds all the credit: metformin is derived from French lilac, a traditional remedy for high blood sugar.

Research shows that for many medical conditions so-called alternative treatments such as herbs and supplements can't compete with conventional drugs. Yet there is no doubt that some of them may be able to influence blood sugar. So should you try an alternative approach if you have diabetes? You may already have done so. In a recent survey published in the *American Journal of Public Health*, 57 per cent of people with diabetes said they had tried complementary and alternative medicine within the previous year, and 34 per cent said they had tried treatments specifically for diabetes. But some of the therapies that may be most promising are relatively little used.

There may be good reasons to be wary. First, when it comes to the licensing of herbal products, up to now the UK has had some of the most pragmatic and liberal laws in the world. This is partly because until 2005 there was no European-wide law regulating the manufacture and sale of herbal medicines. New European Union laws now regulate this important medicinal market by means of the Traditional Herbal Medicinal Products Directive (THMPD), thereby ensuring good quality herbal medicines for over-the-counter sales. To register a product, detailed evidence of safety and quality will be required, but not of efficacy. So clinical trial evidence is not required, but documented proof of medicinal use within Europe has to be submitted. This directive is an important step forward in protecting the health of the public.

In the UK, herbal supplements, while growing in popularity, are still outside the realm of mainstream medicine because

Involve your doctor

Once openly hostile to alternative approaches to medicine, doctors are increasingly accepting that natural approaches sometimes work. A recent study of GPs found that half of them offered access to some form of complementary medicine, and almost one-third provided it in-house. If you decide to try one of the therapies in this chapter, be sure to consult your doctor first. He or she may be able to refer you to a local practitioner, such as a herbalist or acupuncturist. It is also important to keep your doctor informed once you start your therapy.

they are studied less vigorously than drugs are. Still, there are glimmers of potential in the small amount of research that does exist. The therapies covered here are those that show the most promise for helping to control diabetes or some of its major complications. Because they have undergone relatively little research, regimens and doses can only be suggested and should not be taken as medical recommendations. In fact, it's worth repeating that we don't actually *recommend* any of these treatments. If you choose to look into them, the following information may help to guide your choices. Be sure to consult your doctor before embarking on any of the therapies.

Acupuncture

Can you really bring down blood sugar by having your skin poked with thin needles? Practitioners of traditional Chinese medicine (TCM) say yes – but for reasons well outside the realm of Western medicine. According to the philosophy of TCM, diseases arise from imbalances in the flow of life energy, which courses through the body along invisible pathways called meridians. Acupuncture, which involves inserting needles at specific points in the meridian system, is said to bring this energy into balance and improve health. Different points are associated with specific physical functions. Stimulating the pancreas 'acupoint', for example, may increase insulin secretion, while probing the bladder acupoint may help to treat frequent urination.

Western doctors used to dismiss acupuncture completely. It just didn't make sense, especially when the meridian system didn't appear to be related to any obvious part of the anatomy. Nowadays, most people who use acupuncture receive private treatment. Some private health care providers, such as BUPA, PPP and WPA, pay for treatment under their healthcare policies. However, the use of acupuncture within the NHS is growing more rapidly than that of any other complementary therapy. Many physiotherapy departments within NHS hospitals offer acupuncture and more than 2,000 GPs and hospital doctors are trained in acupuncture techniques. NHS Direct lists diabetes as one of the conditions which acupuncture may help to alleviate.

The change in attitude is partly due to rigorous studies in the West that have found that acupuncture can be effective for relieving pain, making it especially promising for people who have neuropathy. A Manchester Royal Infirmary study found that 77 per cent of Type 2 diabetes patients with chronic pain from neuropathy showed significant improvement in their primary and secondary symptoms through acupuncture treatments. In the follow-up period, 67 per cent were able to stop or significantly reduce their medications. How does acupuncture achieve such results? It has been shown that acupoints have denser-than-usual concentrations of nerves, and stimulating them appears to make the brain release natural painkillers.

Whether acupuncture can lower blood sugar is less certain. Most of the research showing an effect on blood sugar has been done in China, where studies do not always comply with Western scientific standards. But a review of several Chinese studies, published in the *Journal of Traditional Chinese Medicine*, found that acupuncture consistently lowered blood sugar in people with diabetes by about 50 per cent. In one of these studies, average blood sugar actually dropped from 21.2mmol/l to 6.5mmol/l after acupuncture treatments.

IF YOU TRY IT Don't expect dramatic blood sugar results. Although the World Health Organization and the British Acupuncture Council recommend acupuncture for a wide variety of problems, Type 2 diabetes and neuropathy do not appear on their lists. Be sure to tell your practitioner if you have neuropathy or poor circulation. The therapist will want to be extra cautious when needling the slow-healing skin of your lower legs and feet.

What happens in an acupuncture treatment? Typically, you will feel a prick, a tingling sensation or a dull ache when needles first go in, but the feeling quickly goes away. Treatment generally involves inserting needles in 4 to 12 acupoints and leaving them there for about 15 to 30 minutes. Once the needles are in place, practitioners often twist or manipulate them by hand to regulate the flow of energy in the body, which produces a dull ache that can be uncomfortable but is thought to be important for releasing chemicals into the nervous system. Needles may also be heated or charged with low-level electrical current.

To find a qualified practitioner in your area, get a list of registered acupuncture practitioners from the British Acupuncture Council (www.medicalacupuncture.org. uk; tel 020 8735 0400).

Herbal treatments

Some of the most promising alternative treatments for high blood sugar come from nature's pharmacy. Plants and herbs have long been part of traditional treatment for diabetes, and of all the alternative treatments they may be the closest to 'real' medicine. In fact, some countries, such as Germany, require doctors to study herbal medicine as part of their medical training. So it is important to respect the potential power of herbs and use them with caution.

Always check with your doctor before using any herbal remedy, even if you are taking it for something other than diabetes. Many herbs can affect blood pressure and liver function, and they may interfere with medications that you are taking. If you take herbal supplements it is essential to monitor your blood sugar closely in order to guard against hypoglycaemia, help your doctor to decide on changes in your drug treatment, and to tell if the supplement is working. If it is, remember that no natural remedy can replace medication or insulin, even if it allows you to reduce their dosages.

GYMNEMA: THE SUGAR BUSTER

A woody plant found in tropical forests in India and Africa, *Gymnema sylvestre* has been used for centuries as a remedy for diabetes. Its name in Hindi is *gurmar*, or 'sugar destroyer', and chewing its leaves is said to take away your taste for sweetness. Laboratory analyses have found that gymnema boosts the activity of enzymes that help cells to take up glucose, so there is less of it floating in the blood. More than a decade ago, animal studies found that gymnema lowers blood sugar – but not in animals that had had their pancreases removed. These findings led researchers to theorize that gymnema may battle high blood sugar by:

- Boosting the release of insulin by making cells in the pancreas more permeable
- Stimulating insulin-making beta cells in the pancreas
- Increasing the number of beta cells

Does it work in people? Herbalists believe that if any herb will bring down your blood sugar, it's gymnema, but there is a shortage of controlled studies to confirm that assertion. In one study from a medical institute in India, Type 2 diabetes patients who took gymnema in addition to medication reduced their average blood sugar levels more than a control group who took only the drug. About a quarter of those taking gymnema were able to stop their medication completely. Similar results have been seen in research on people with Type 1 diabetes.

IF YOU TRY IT Expect an effect – and be sure to inform your doctor so he or she can coordinate your herb doses and the rest of your treatment. Safety studies have not been done on gymnema, but it has a long history and no known reports of unpleasant side effects. The lack of data makes gymnema inappropriate for women who are pregnant or breastfeeding. Beyond that, the main concern is that blood sugar may fall too low, especially if the herb is taken with a diabetes medication.

How good is the proof?

While there may be thousands of satisfied users of an alternative therapy, in the eyes of science it cannot be considered effective until carefully conducted studies have proved it to be. Why are researchers such sticklers? This is what they look for.

▸ **Studies in which people in one group get the real treatment and people in a control group get a dummy treatment (placebo).** Without a control group, some people may feel better (or say that they do) simply because they expect to – or because improvements are really due to something other than the treatment.

▸ **Studies in which neither participants nor researchers know who is getting the real thing and who is getting the placebo.** That is another way to make sure that positive results are due to the treatment and not to any expectations from subjects who have been tipped off, perhaps by researchers themselves.

▸ **Studies that involve large numbers of people.** This is to make sure that the results are not a fluke, are published in respected journals and are reviewed by experts to make sure that the research is rigorous.

FENUGREEK: A POTENT SPICE

Although probably best known as a spice and flavour enhancer from the Mediterranean and Near East, fenugreek has a long tradition of medicinal uses. Early Greek and Roman catalogues of medicines list it as a treatment for high blood sugar. Animal research and a handful of small human studies suggest that it may indeed be an effective treatment. In one study, for example, 60 people with Type 2 diabetes who took a total of 25g of fenugreek powder in two equal doses at lunch and dinner over a six-month period lowered their fasting blood sugar from an average of 8.3mmol/l to 6.2mmol/l.

Fenugreek seems to slow digestion, hinder the absorption of carbohydrates and put the brakes on the movement of glucose through the body. All this may be because fenugreek is a legume – a relative of lentils, chickpeas, geen peas and peanuts – and is rich in fibre. But laboratory studies also indicate that fenugreek contains an amino acid shown to boost the release of insulin.

IF YOU TRY IT Fenugreek rides a fine line between being a supplement or a food. In one study, volunteers took their daily doses by eating defatted (where the fat has been removed) fenugreek seed powder, which has a mild, nutty taste, in unleavened bread. You can also make tea by soaking the seeds in cold water. Another way to consume it is to mix fenugreek seed powder with vegetables or fruit in a blender to make a smoothie. Adding fenugreek to your diet is the ideal way to obtain it, because taking therapeutic doses in capsules can mean swallowing a lot of pills.

Although it can cause flatulence and diarrhoea, fenugreek is generally considered safe; in rare instances, people have had severe reactions to it. You should avoid fenugreek if you are pregnant or breastfeeding or have liver or kidney disease. Never take it within 2 hours of taking a diabetes medication, as it may interfere with your body's absorption of the drug. You should also be cautious if you are taking blood thinners, as fenugreek may interact with them.

Bitter melon

A dietary staple in India and Asia, bitter melon, known as karella in the UK, is in fact a vegetable. It has long been a folk remedy for diabetes in the East and studies in humans suggest that it may help to lower blood sugar. In one study, 100 people with Type 2 diabetes found their blood sugar fell significantly hours after drinking its unpalatable pulp. Karela contains plant insulin, thought to help cells to use glucose, and other substances that block intestinal sugar absorption. It should not be taken during pregnancy. Pending formal studies, Diabetes UK does not recommend taking Karela capsules.

GINSENG: THE CURE-ALL

Ginseng refers to three different plants. *Panax ginseng* (known as Asian, Chinese or Korean ginseng) has been used for thousands of years in traditional Chinese medicine to enhance longevity, revitalize the body and to treat a host of ailments. American ginseng (*Panax quinquefolius*) is a close cousin, while Siberian ginseng (*Eleutherococcus senticosus*) is only distantly related.

Ginseng's genus name, Panax, comes from two Greek words for 'cure' and 'all' and the herb is reputed to help build resistance to disease, aid recovery from illness, combat the physical effects of stress and even promote longer life but this reputation has yet to be verified by research. Experts agree that it contains compounds called ginsenosides (whose functions are unclear) and that *Panax ginseng* also contains panaxans, substances that can lower blood sugar. Research into ginseng's effects on diabetes is inconclusive, but a University of Toronto study, published in a respected medical journal, found that taking 3g of American ginseng 40 minutes before eating lowered blood sugar by about 20 per cent compared with a control group.

Although it is still unclear how ginseng works to bring down blood sugar levels, animal studies suggest that it may slow carbohydrate absorption or boost cells' uptake of glucose. Most research so far has been done on ginseng root. But a recent study on mice bred to develop diabetes found that an extract of ginseng berry, which has different concentrations of ginsenosides, lowered blood sugar levels and improved insulin sensitivity.

IF YOU TRY IT *Panax ginseng* and Siberian ginseng are available in extract form but the herb is traditionally consumed in teas. Look for tea bags containing the powdered root, which are sometimes labelled as 'red ginseng'. Be sure to consult your doctor before trying ginseng. Do not take ginseng during pregnancy, or if you are suffering from obesity, insomnia or high blood pressure.

Nutrient micromanagement

All those vegetables you are eating on the 10 Per Cent Plan will provide with you with plenty of micronutrients. Despite that, some micronutrients may be worth taking in supplement form when you have Type 2 diabetes.

The body needs only very small amounts of micronutrients, but they have powerful, if often subtle, effects. Many are involved with metabolism, and even a moderate deficiency in these may contribute to chronic diseases. Getting more of certain micronutrients appears to help control diabetes. People with diabetes may be low in some of these because frequent urination may flush them from the body quickly.

It can be difficult to work out if you are deficient in certain micronutrients because relatively little is known about them. But it makes sense to take a daily multivitamin to provide you with at least the minimum amounts you need to keep healthy. Beyond that, supplemental doses of specific micronutrients that are not found in most multivitamins may help to keep your blood glucose under better control.

CONTROL WITH **CHROMIUM**

The trace mineral chromium is essential for growth and good health. It also helps the body to maintain normal blood glucose levels by using insulin efficiently. For example, chromium appears to make it easier for insulin to bind with cells so that glucose can enter tissues rather than building up in the blood. Do you get enough chromium? The Food Standards Agency states that adults need at least 0.025mg or 25mcg of chromium a day. Good dietary sources are meat, cheese, vegetables, wholegrains, wine and beer. A varied and balanced diet should provide all the chromium you need.

Will getting more chromium help with blood sugar control? Even though it is one of the better known micronutrients suggested for diabetes, research with people who have high blood sugar has produced mixed results. In one of the largest studies, 180 people were assigned to groups that were given either chromium (two different doses were tried) or a placebo. Those given the chromium significantly reduced their A1C numbers (which indicate long-term blood sugar control) after four months, and those given the highest dose (1,000mcg) lowered their cholesterol too. Several studies have shown similar results, but in some others chromium either had no effect on blood sugar or the findings were ambiguous.

You may have heard that chromium helps the body to lose fat without losing muscle, and some research points in that direction. In one study of 122 moderately overweight people, those who took 400mcg of chromium a day saw an average weight loss of nearly 3kg (6lb 3oz) over three months. But few other studies have backed these findings.

Garlic for the heart

Diabetes is linked to heart disease, which has its own arsenal of herbal medicines, the most important of which is garlic. This has been shown to reduce 'bad' LDL cholesterol by about 16 per cent and to lower blood pressure. In one study, garlic trimmed plaque by about 3 per cent in the arteries of people who took it. And some studies find that garlic lowers blood sugar as well. Just be sure you don't take garlic if you are taking a blood thinner (it will thin your blood even more), and don't cook it if you want medicinal benefits, because heat changes its chemistry. The best way to tap garlic's powers is to eat it raw – then stay at home for the night.

IF YOU TRY IT The biggest blood sugar benefits have been seen in people who have a low-chromium diet, which typically includes lots of sugar and refined white flour – low-chromium foods that actually trigger chromium loss. Since you are already avoiding those foods on the 10 Per Cent Plan, you're ahead of the game from the start.

If you take a chromium supplement – and Diabetes UK advises doing so only when a chromium deficiency has been diagnosed – do not exceed the safe level of 10mg a day. Chromium is a heavy metal, and large doses may build up in the body, potentially leading to kidney damage. Chromium comes in different forms. Most studies use chromium picolinate, which the body absorbs better than chromium chloride.

OTHER POSSIBLE BLOOD-SUGAR BUSTERS

A number of other plant-based supplements have been suggested as blood-sugar busters, based on preliminary research that is even thinner than that for the supplements discussed above. They include the following.

BILBERRY Related to the blueberry and grown in Europe and Canada, bilberry is a folk remedy for diabetes although no human studies have been done on its blood-sugar effects. In animals it has been shown to lower blood glucose by 26 per cent and triglycerides by 39 per cent, potentially making it even more beneficial if you have heart disease. The safety of the extract has not been established (high doses may interact with blood thinners), but it is quite safe to eat as a fruit.

PRICKLY PEAR Also known as nopal, this cactus is a Mexican folk remedy for diabetes and has been studied in small, uncontrolled trials. In two of them, people with Type 2 diabetes who consumed 500g (just over 1lb) of nopal saw their blood sugar drop significantly within a few hours. One reason for this may be prickly pear's high fibre content. Possible side effects include gastrointestinal distress.

PTEROCARPUS MARSUPIUM The bark of this tree from India contains a compound called epicatechin, that some sudies have found improves the function of insulin-producing beta cells in the pancreas. In one study from India of 97 people with Type 2 diabetes, 69 per cent of those taking 2 to 4g of the herb daily achieved good glucose control within 12 weeks.

Help for nerve damage

No supplement or therapy is going to cure you of neuropathy, but if you have the irritation, pain and tingling of this common diabetes complication, even a little bit of relief can make a big difference. Because nerve damage can affect so many aspects of your health (including your sense of touch and pain, sexual function and digestion), it is important to prevent high blood sugar from causing more harm. If you are doing everything you can with diet, exercise, and medical treatments, it may be time to look into other options.

THE ALLURE OF **Alpha-Lipoic Acid**

What causes diabetic neuropathy? One theory is that neuropathy begins when nerve cells swell. If you trace reasons for the swelling back several steps, it appears that glucose teams up with an enzyme to draw water into cells and not let it out. That's where alpha-lipoic acid (ALA) comes in. This powerful antioxidant is thought to block the enzyme that leads to swelling. Furthermore, ALA protects cells against the damaging effects of free radicals – destructive molecules that are also thought to play a role in nerve damage.

The body makes small amounts of ALA, and you derive a bit more from foods such as spinach, but these sources don't provide enough to do battle against neuropathy. For that, you need a supplement. Can ALA help people with nerve damage to feel better? Many believe it can and researchers have looked into ALA more rigorously than they have most other alternative therapies.

While results are still not conclusive, they have been encouraging. In one trial involving 328 people with Type 2 diabetes, those who received ALA injections daily for three weeks felt significantly less pain from neuropathy than those who didn't receive the treatment. An even larger follow-up trial, however, failed to find much of an effect from ALA.

In order to assess the balance of evidence, researchers at a German diabetes institute recently reviewed four different well-controlled studies and found that, on average, people's neuropathy symptoms improved steadily while they were taking ALA. Studies in the United States, including one at the Mayo Clinic, have produced similar results.

IF YOU TRY IT Some of the best studies have used injected ALA, but there is evidence that pills can help to control neuropathy, too, with suggested doses ranging from 100 to 600mg. Apart from rare allergic reactions such as skin rashes, few serious safety issues have arisen with ALA in 30 years of testing and clinical use for neuropathy in Germany. However, it has been shown to be toxic in animals with a thiamin deficiency, so it may be worth taking ALA in conjunction with a thiamin supplement or multivitamin.

MAGNETS: A POSITIVE FORCE?

The idea of easing nerve symptoms by putting magnets in your shoes or lying on a magnetic mattress may strike you as wacky, but is it? After all, magnetic fields are involved in plenty of processes in the body, from cell division to transmitting signals through the nervous system. In fact, a century ago, magnets were a popular form of medicine and were often used to treat pain. Today, such ideas are far from mainstream, but they may be worth a second look.

One of the most intriguing studies on magnet therapy involved people with chronic neuropathic foot pain. In the study (conducted by a sceptical New York neurologist), when 19 people wore magnetic insoles in their shoes for four months, 75 per cent reported feeling significant relief. In a recent follow-up study with a group of 375 people, the researcher repeated the experiment. The study found that magnets improved a range of symptoms, including burning, tingling, numbness and pain. The researchers concluded that magnets affect the firing of pain receptors in the skin. It has also been suggested that magnets draw blood into areas that need more oxygen by attracting the iron in it and they help blood vessel walls to relax by influencing the flow of ions.

IF YOU TRY THEM The benefits of magnets are still far from proven, but using them appears to be harmless – with a few caveats. For example, don't use magnets if you have a pacemaker, and avoid using magnets on your head or in the area of cancer tumours or infections. There are no standards for how strong magnets should be to treat neuropathy, but products such as magnetic insoles are widely available. Look for therapeutic magnets at a health products store or search online under 'magnetic health products'.

suc

cess

(suc•cess) *noun*

1. A favourable outcome or result.

2. The attainment of wealth, status or fame.

3. Better diabetes control. The logs in this chapter will help you to track to your success on the 10 Per Cent Plan, and the recipes help you to produce delicious meals.

PART FOUR

Resources

Tools and recipes for
success

In this book you've discovered how making gradual changes to your daily routine can trigger a seismic shift towards better diabetes control. To help ensure your success, we've provided the following resources.

Use these logs to monitor your progress on the 10 Per Cent Plan and these recipes to facilitate your menu planning.

Tracking your efforts is important. Don't rely on your general impressions of what you eat and how much you exercise: write it down. Seeing the truth in black and white will reveal pitfalls and inspire you to build on your efforts. And watching your weight and blood sugar numbers go down will make it all worth while.

To ensure that they do go down, you will probably want to follow some of the Plate Approach menu suggestions in Step Three. To help you, we have supplied recipes for some of those dishes here, along with many others. Remember, any food is allowed, but portion control is always essential.

Personal contract

Keep this contract as a reminder of your commitment.

I vow that over the next six months, I will learn and implement the six steps to better diabetes control presented in the 10 Per Cent Plan.

My goals
Intermediate weight-loss: _____
Ultimate target weight: _____

My strategies
To reach these goals, I agree to:
1. Eat breakfast and small snacks so that I never allow myself to become too hungry.
2. Follow the Plate Approach at every meal.
3. Limit my food portions.
4. Master the following 'disaster' foods by modifying recipes and/or eating smaller portions.

_____

_____

_____

5. Build up to 45 minutes of walking most days of the week.
6. Practise one stress-relief approach every day.

To track my progress, I agree to monitor and record my blood sugar regularly.

My reminders
Why I want to do all that I can to control my diabetes:
1. _____
2. _____
3. _____

Signed: _____
Date: _____

Food diary

Photocopy this form seven times, or duplicate the columns in a notebook. For one week, carry the log with you wherever you go and write down everything you eat or drink, noting the time, portion size (use the guide on page 85 to help you estimate this) and any relevant notes, such as the circumstances or what you were feeling at the time. Use nutrition labels to find out the calorie content of packaged foods. To estimate calories for fresh foods, refer to a calorie-counter book or log on to www.weightlossresources.co.uk/calories/calorie_counter.htm

TIME	WHAT I ATE	PORTION	NOTES	CALORIES

Activity log

Every time you do something active, note it on this form. That includes going for your daily walk and doing Sugar-Buster exercises, 30-second Fitness Boosters or the Day's-End Wind-Down. Also include activities such as gardening. Record the minutes spent, and add up the number at the end of the day.

	TIME	ACTIVITY	MINUTES
MONDAY			
		MONDAY TOTAL	
TUESDAY			
		TUESDAY TOTAL	
WEDNESDAY			
		WEDNESDAY TOTAL	
THURSDAY			
		THURSDAY TOTAL	
FRIDAY			
		FRIDAY TOTAL	
SATURDAY			
		SATURDAY TOTAL	
SUNDAY			
		SUNDAY TOTAL	
		WEEKLY TOTAL	

Results tracker

Use this form to keep track of how well you are doing on the 10 Per Cent Plan. Start each day by writing down your morning weight. Then, at the end of the day, consider all the elements of the plan. Did you have breakfast and eat regularly throughout the day? Eat plenty of vegetables and limit high-calorie foods? Eat reasonable portions? Get some exercise? Manage stress well?

After reviewing your performance in each area, give yourself an overall letter grade (A, B, C, D or E) for the day. Write a brief explanation of why you gave yourself that grade. As days go by, compare your grades with your weight patterns and use your notes to find areas in which you can improve.

DATE	WEIGHT	GRADE	REASON FOR MY GRADE

Blood sugar log

Ask your doctor how often you should check your blood glucose level, based on your personal health situation. Use your own blood sugar log, or copy this form and fill in the appropriate columns. Be sure to save the readings in a file folder. You will want to look back on them to see how much you improve on the 10 Per Cent Plan.

DATE	DAY	BREAKFAST	LUNCH	DINNER	BEDTIME
	MONDAY				
	TUESDAY				
	WEDNESDAY				
	THURSDAY				
	FRIDAY				
	SATURDAY				
	SUNDAY				
	MONDAY				
	TUESDAY				
	WEDNESDAY				
	THURSDAY				
	FRIDAY				
	SATURDAY				
	SUNDAY				
	MONDAY				
	TUESDAY				
	WEDNESDAY				
	THURSDAY				
	FRIDAY				
	SATURDAY				
	SUNDAY				
	MONDAY				
	TUESDAY				
	WEDNESDAY				
	THURSDAY				
	FRIDAY				
	SATURDAY				
	SUNDAY				

Healthy Recipes

Steak roulade with spinach, carrots and pepper

SERVES 6

125ml (4fl oz) red wine

5 tablespoons reduced-sodium soy sauce

2 tablespoons caster sugar

1 teaspoon finely chopped garlic

675g (1½lb) thick flank steak, butterflied

175g (6oz) fresh baby spinach leaves

4 spring onions, coarsely chopped

⅛ teaspoon salt

450g (1lb) carrots, grated

1 jar (about 350g) roasted red peppers, well drained

1. Combine the wine, soy sauce, sugar and garlic in a large resealable plastic bag or other container. Add the steak and turn to coat. Marinate in the refrigerator for at least 2 hours and up to 4 hours.

2. Meanwhile, rinse the spinach, leaving some water clinging to the leaves. Cook in a large saucepan over a moderate heat, stirring frequently, for about 1 minute or until just wilted. Drain and transfer to a plate to cool.

3. Preheat the oven to 190°C (375°F, gas mark 5). Remove the steak from the marinade and pat dry. Set the marinade aside. Spread the spinach in an even layer over the steak. Top with the spring onions and sprinkle with the salt. Layer the carrots on top, then the peppers. Starting at a long side, roll up tightly to enclose the filling. Secure the roll in several places with wooden cocktail sticks. Place the roll, seam side down, in a shallow tin and brush all over with the marinade.

4. Roast for 15 minutes, then spoon any pan juices on top of the roll. Roast for a further 20 minutes for medium-rare, or until cooked to taste. Allow to rest for 10 minutes.

5. Meanwhile, boil the remaining marinade in a small saucepan just until thick enough to coat a spoon. Strain and set aside.

6. Cut the roll diagonally into 5mm (¼in) slices. Drizzle a little marinade on each plate and top with the slices.

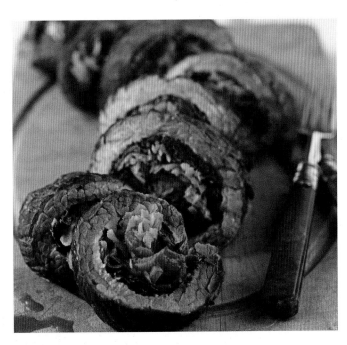

NUTRITIONAL INFORMATION
PER SERVING: 324kcal, 27g protein, 18g carbohydrate, 14g fat, 4g saturated fat, 65mg cholesterol, 4g fibre, 473mg sodium

Braised ham with sweet potatoes and apples

SERVES 4

1 tablespoon Dijon mustard

1 tablespoon finely chopped
   fresh ginger

½ teaspoon ground cloves

225ml (8fl oz) plus
   1 tablespoon apple juice

1 large sweet potato, peeled
   and cut into 3mm (⅛in)
   slices

450g (1lb) lean ham steak

1 Granny Smith apple,
   peeled, cored and cut into
   12 wedges

1 tablespoon cornflour

50g (1¾oz) spring onions,
   diagonally sliced into fine
   strips

1. Stir together the mustard, ginger, cloves and 225ml (8fl oz) of the apple juice in a large frying pan. Bring to a simmer, then add the sweet potato. Cover tightly and simmer for 15 minutes.

2. Add the ham steak and cover with the sweet potato slices. Arrange the apple wedges on top. Cover and simmer for 10–15 minutes or until the apple and sweet potato are tender and the ham is heated through.

3. Meanwhile, stir together the cornflour and the remaining apple juice in a small bowl until well blended.

4. With a slotted spoon, transfer the ham, sweet potato and apple to a platter. Cover with foil to keep warm.

5. Stir a little of the hot pan juices into the cornflour mixture until smooth. Add to the rest of the juice in the pan and cook, stirring, over a moderate heat for 1 minute or until slightly thickened.

6. Divide the ham, sweet potato and apples among four plates. Spoon over the sauce and garnish with the onions.

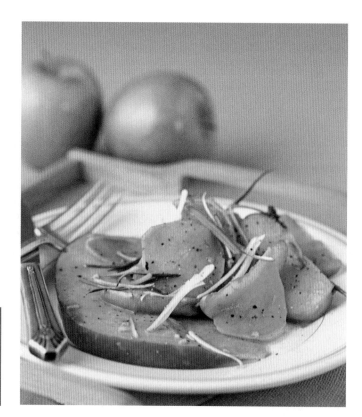

NUTRITIONAL INFORMATION

PER SERVING: 264kcal,
21g protein, 26g carbohydrate,
9g fat, 3g saturated fat,
25mg cholesterol, 2g fibre,
1123mg sodium

Pork fillet with honey-mustard sauce

SERVES 4

1 tablespoon chopped fresh
  rosemary or
  1 teaspoon dried

2 garlic cloves, crushed

1 teaspoon grated lemon
  zest

½ teaspoon salt

1 pork fillet, about 450g
  (1lb), trimmed of all visible
  fat

5 tablespoons fresh lemon
  juice

4 tablespoons clear honey

3 tablespoons coarse-grain
  Dijon mustard

125ml (4fl oz) reduced-fat
  single cream

1 tablespoon plain flour

1. Preheat the oven to 200°C (400°F, gas mark 6). Line a small roasting tin with foil.

2. Stir together the rosemary, garlic, lemon zest and salt in a small bowl. Rub evenly over the pork, then place the pork in the tin.

3. Stir together the lemon juice, honey and mustard in a small bowl. Transfer half of the sauce to a small saucepan and set aside.

4. Brush the pork with 2 tablespoons of the remaining sauce. Roast, basting two or three times with sauce, for about 25 minutes or until glazed and golden brown.

5. Meanwhile, pour the cream into a small bowl and whisk in the flour until smooth. Warm the reserved sauce over low heat. Gradually whisk in the cream mixture and cook, whisking constantly, for about 3 minutes or until thick. Serve with the pork.

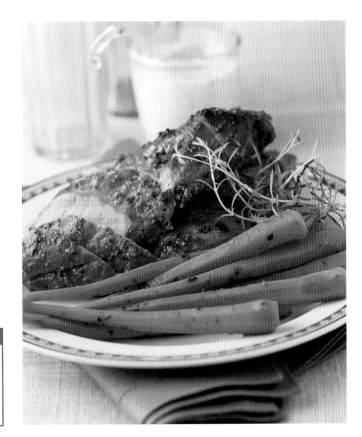

NUTRITIONAL INFORMATION

PER SERVING: 249kcal,
26g protein, 17g carbohydrate,
9g fat, 4g saturated fat,
70mg cholesterol, 1g fibre,
292mg sodium

Garden beef stir-fry with hoisin sauce

SERVES 4

350g (12oz) lean sirloin
steak

2 tablespoons teriyaki sauce

10 shiitake mushrooms

225g (8oz) sugarsnap peas
or mange touts

2 large red peppers

3 tablespoons hoisin sauce

2 tablespoons cornflour

300ml (½ pint) chicken stock
made without salt

3 teaspoons vegetable oil

4 spring onions, thinly sliced
on the diagonal

2 garlic cloves, crushed

1. To make slicing easier, chill the steak in the freezer for
20 minutes. Cut across the grain into strips about 3mm
(⅛in) thick, then halve extra-long pieces crossways.
Toss with the teriyaki sauce in a medium bowl. Marinate
in the refrigerator for at least 15 minutes and ideally for
several hours.

2. Meanwhile, remove the stalks from the mushrooms and
thinly slice the caps. Trim the ends from the peas and
remove the strings. Cut the peppers into thin strips. Stir
together the hoisin sauce, cornflour and 4 tablespoons of
the stock in a small bowl until smooth. Set aside.

3. Heat 1 teaspoon of the oil in a large non-stick frying pan
or wok over a high heat until hot but not smoking. Add
the spring onions and stir-fry for 1 minute. Transfer to a
large bowl. Add the steak and garlic to the pan and stir-
fry for 2 minutes or until the meat is no longer pink.
Transfer to the bowl. Add another 1 teaspoon of the oil
and the mushrooms to the pan. Stir-fry for 3 minutes or
until they begin to soften, then transfer to the bowl.
Add the remaining 1 teaspoon of oil with the peas and
peppers. Stir-fry for 1–2 minutes or until they soften.

4. Return the meat and vegetables to the pan and stir in the
remaining stock. Cover and cook over moderate heat for
2–3 minutes or until the ingredients are heated through
and the vegetables are just tender. Whisk the hoisin sauce
mixture and add to the pan. Stir-fry until the sauce boils,
then cook for a further 1 minute.

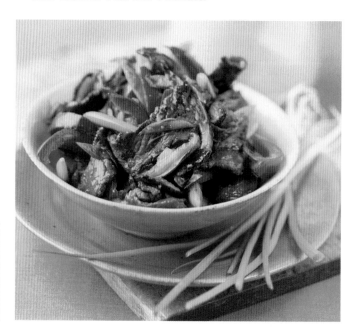

NUTRITIONAL INFORMATION

PER SERVING: 250kcal,
7g protein, 19g carbohydrate,
8g fat, 2g saturated fat,
44mg cholesterol, 3g fibre,
1075mg sodium

Barbecued chicken

SERVES 6

1½ teaspoons olive oil

1 medium onion, chopped

2 garlic cloves, crushed

1 can (about 400g) tomatoes in passata or purée

5 tablespoons pineapple juice

4 tablespoons water

2 tablespoons soft brown sugar

2 tablespoons light soy sauce

1 tablespoon coarse-grain Dijon mustard

1 teaspoon dried thyme

½ teaspoon salt

¼ teaspoon hickory-flavoured liquid smoke (optional)

675g (1½lb) chicken breasts, skin removed

675g (1½lb) chicken thighs and drumsticks, skin removed

1. Prepare the barbecue for a medium fire (or heat the grill). Coat the rack with vegetable oil.

2. Heat the oil in a medium saucepan over a moderately high heat. Sauté the onion and garlic for 5 minutes or until softened. Stir in the tomatoes, pineapple juice, water, brown sugar, soy sauce, mustard, thyme, salt and liquid smoke, if using. Reduce the heat to moderate, cover and simmer for 5 minutes.

3. Transfer the sauce to a food processor or blender and purée until smooth. Return to the saucepan and simmer, whisking frequently, for about 5 minutes or until slightly thickened. Set aside half of the sauce.

4. Brush the chicken pieces on both sides with sauce, then barbecue or grill for 15 minutes, basting with sauce and turning the chicken halfway through cooking. Continue cooking, without basting, for about 15 minutes or until no longer pink and the juices run clear. Reheat the reserved sauce to serve with the chicken.

NUTRITIONAL INFORMATION

PER SERVING: 256kcal, 42g protein, 10g carbohydrate, 6g fat, 1g saturated fat, 148mg cholesterol, 0.7g fibre, 676mg sodium

---

Chicken Marsala

SERVES 4

4 skinless chicken breast fillets, 115–175g (4–6oz) each

1 onion, chopped

1 teaspoon chopped garlic

175ml (6fl oz) Marsala wine

2 cans (about 400g each) chopped tomatoes

¼ teaspoon freshly ground black pepper

2 tablespoons chopped parsley

1 tablespoon chopped fresh basil or 1 teaspoon dried

2–3 tablespoons freshly grated Parmesan cheese (optional)

1. Spray a large frying pan with cooking spray. Add the chicken and cook over a moderate heat, turning to brown on all sides. Add the onion and garlic and cook until lightly browned. Increase the heat to high, add the wine and cook until completely reduced. Remove the chicken.

2. Reduce the heat to moderate again and add the tomatoes, pepper, parsley and basil. Simmer, stirring occasionally, for about 30 minutes or until the sauce begins to thicken. Return the chicken fillets to the pan and cook until they are heated through.

3. Sprinkle with the cheese, if using, then serve.

Note: This is delicious served over boiled noodles. Other vegetables, such as mushrooms, courgettes, green pepper and broccoli, can be added for variety.

NUTRITIONAL INFORMATION

PER SERVING: 240kcal, 32g protein, 11g carbohydrate, 4g fat, 2g saturated fat, 87mg cholesterol, 2g fibre, 216mg sodium

Greek chicken with capers

SERVES 4

4 skinless chicken breast fillets, 115g (4oz) each

2 tablespoons plain flour

2 tablespoons seasoned dried breadcrumbs

1 teaspoon dried oregano

1 tablespoon olive oil

125g (4oz) thinly sliced onion

3 garlic cloves, crushed

225ml (8fl oz) chicken stock made without salt

125ml (4fl oz) white wine (optional)

2 tablespoons lemon juice

2 tablespoons capers

25g (1oz) feta cheese, crumbled

4 black olives, chopped (optional)

1. Pound the chicken fillets to an even thickness between two sheets of greaseproof paper. Combine the flour, breadcrumbs and oregano in a shallow bowl or plate, then coat the chicken in the mixture.

2. Heat the oil in a large non-stick frying pan over a moderate heat. Add the chicken and brown on both sides, then remove from the pan. Add the onion and garlic and sauté for 2 minutes. Stir in the stock, wine and lemon juice and bring to the boil. Return the chicken to the pan, reduce the heat and simmer for about 10 minutes or until no longer pink and the juices run clear. Sprinkle with the capers and cheese, cover and heat gently until the cheese softens. Top with the olives, if using.

NUTRITIONAL INFORMATION

PER SERVING: 255kcal, 30g protein, 15g carbohydrate, 7g fat, 2g saturated fat, 108mg cholesterol, 1g fibre, 238mg sodium

Tex-Mex turkey casserole

SERVES 6

1 tablespoon vegetable oil

1 onion, coarsely chopped

1 tablespoon mild chilli powder

½ teaspoon ground cinnamon

¼ teaspoon salt

3 tablespoons plain flour

1 can (about 400g) chopped tomatoes

225ml (8fl oz) chicken stock, made without salt

225g (8oz) roast turkey, in a slice 1cm (½in) thick, cut into cubes

2 courgettes, cut into 1cm (½in) cubes

150g (5½oz) frozen sweet-corn kernels

225g (8oz) cooked long-grain white rice

115g (4oz) reduced-fat Cheddar cheese, grated

1. Preheat the oven to 180°C (350°F, gas mark 4).

2. Heat the oil in a large saucepan over a moderate heat. Add the onion and sauté for about 5 minutes or until softened. Stir in the chilli powder, cinnamon, salt and flour. Cook, stirring, for 2 minutes. Stir in the tomatoes and stock and cook, stirring, for about 2 minutes or until slightly thickened.

3. Remove from the heat and stir in the turkey, courgettes, sweetcorn and rice. Pour into a baking dish. (The casserole can be prepared ahead to this point.) Bake for about 40 minutes or until bubbly.

4. Sprinkle with the grated cheese and bake for a further 5 minutes or until melted. Allow to stand for 5 minutes before serving.

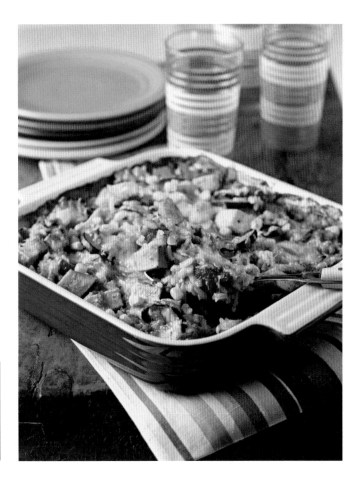

NUTRITIONAL INFORMATION

PER SERVING: 265kcal, 20g protein, 26g carbohydrate, 8g fat, 3g saturated fat, 40mg cholesterol, 1.5g fibre, 257mg sodium

Prawn and vegetable stir-fry

SERVES 4

150ml (¼ pint) water

5 tablespoons low-sodium soy sauce

3 tablespoons white wine or orange juice

2 tablespoons cornflour

1½ teaspoons grated fresh ginger

1 tablespoon vegetable oil

2 garlic cloves, crushed

450g (1lb) raw king prawns, peeled and deveined

400g (14oz) broccoli florets

1 large red pepper, deseeded and cut into strips

1 large yellow pepper, deseeded and cut into strips

115g (4oz) mange tout

85g (3oz) baby corn

125g (4oz) sliced canned water chestnuts

4 spring onions, cut diagonally into 5cm (2in) pieces

1. Stir together the water, soy sauce, wine or orange juice, cornflour and ginger in a small bowl until smooth. Set aside.

2. Heat the oil in a large wok or large, deep frying pan over a moderately high heat until hot. Add the garlic and stir-fry for 1 minute. Add the prawns and stir-fry for about 3 minutes or until pink, then remove with a slotted spoon. Add the broccoli and stir-fry for 2 minutes. Add the peppers, mange tout and baby corn, and stir-fry for another 2 minutes or until just tender.

3. Return the prawns to the wok. Add the water chestnuts and spring onions. Pour in the soy sauce mixture and stir-fry for 1 minute or until the sauce thickens and boils. Serve immediately.

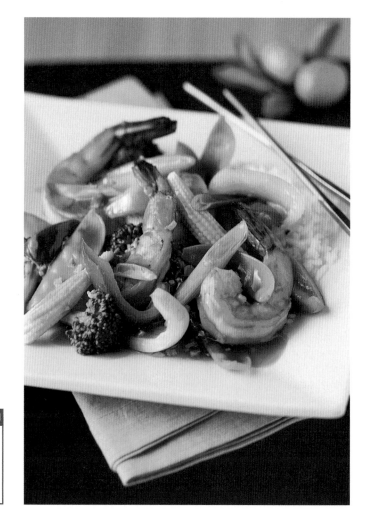

NUTRITIONAL INFORMATION

PER SERVING: 251kcal, 23g protein, 18g carbohydrate, 5g fat, 1g saturated fat, 315mg cholesterol, 5g fibre, 1384mg sodium

Crab and artichoke rice

SERVES 6

1 tablespoon olive oil

3 garlic cloves, crushed

½ green pepper, deseeded and chopped

1 onion, chopped

2 tablespoons chopped parsley

350ml (12fl oz) tomato-based pasta sauce

1 can (about 400g) artichoke hearts, drained (liquid reserved) and quartered

30 black olives, pitted

225g (8oz) crabmeat

400g (14oz) hot, cooked brown or white rice

1. Heat the oil in a large frying pan. Add the garlic, pepper and onion, and sauté until softened.

2. Add the parsley, pasta sauce, artichokes (with liquid), olives and crabmeat.

3. Cook over a moderate heat until hot, stirring occasionally. Fold in the hot cooked rice.

NUTRITIONAL INFORMATION

PER SERVING: 235kcal, 12g protein, 31g carbohydrate, 7g fat ,1g saturated fat, 27mg cholesterol, 2g fibre, 400mg sodium

Baked cod with rocket

SERVES 4

450g (1lb) new potatoes, cut into 1cm (½in) slices

1 onion, thinly sliced

1 tablespoon olive oil

½ teaspoon salt

4 plum tomatoes, deseeded and coarsely chopped

3 garlic cloves, crushed

½ teaspoon dried oregano, crumbled

150g (5½oz) rocket

450g (1lb) cod or halibut fillet, cut into 5cm (2in) chunks

1. Preheat the oven to 180°C (350°F, gas mark 4).

2. Combine the potatoes, onion, oil and ¼ teaspoon of the salt in a large baking dish. Spread out evenly, then bake for 20 minutes, stirring once.

3. Stir in the tomatoes, garlic and oregano. Spread the rocket in an even layer on top. Arrange the fish on the rocket and sprinkle with the remaining ¼ teaspoon salt. Cover with foil and bake for 15–18 minutes or until the fish is just cooked through. Transfer to plates and spoon the pan juices over each serving.

NUTRITIONAL INFORMATION

PER SERVING: 225kcal, 24g protein, 24g carbohydrate, 4.5g fat, 1g saturated fat, 52mg cholesterol, 5g fibre, 336mg sodium

Couscous-stuffed peppers

SERVES 6

6 large peppers (any colour)

1 tablespoon vegetable oil

1 courgette, finely chopped

2 garlic cloves, finely chopped

1 tablespoon fresh lemon juice

400g (14oz) cooked or soaked couscous

1 can (about 400g) chickpeas, drained and rinsed

1 ripe tomato, deseeded and finely chopped

1 teaspoon dried oregano, crumbled

½ teaspoon salt

¼ teaspoon freshly ground black pepper

50g (1¾oz) feta cheese, crumbled

1. Slice the tops off the peppers and reserve. Scoop out the membranes and seeds, and discard. Simmer the peppers and tops, covered, in a large saucepan of lightly salted boiling water for 5 minutes. Drain.

2. Preheat the oven to 180°C (350°F, gas mark 4). Heat the oil in a medium saucepan over a moderate heat. Add the courgette and garlic, and sauté for 2 minutes. Stir in the lemon juice. Cook for 1 minute, then remove from the heat. Stir in the couscous, chickpeas, tomato, oregano, salt and pepper. Stir in the cheese.

3. Fill each pepper with the couscous mixture and place upright in a shallow baking dish. Cover with the pepper tops. Bake for about 20 minutes or just until the filling is heated through.

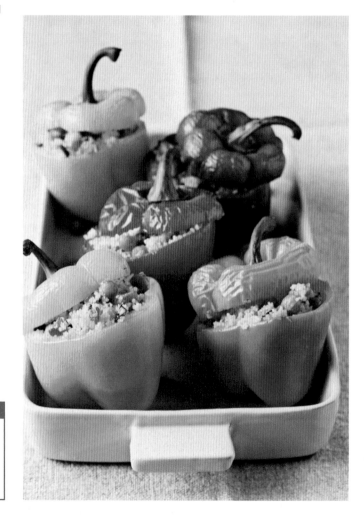

NUTRITIONAL INFORMATION

PER SERVING: 205kcal, 8g protein, 36g carbohydrate, 6g fat, 2g saturated fat, 6mg cholesterol, 5g fibre, 401mg sodium

Tuna salad Provençale

SERVES 4

55g (2oz) green beans

225g (8oz) mixed salad greens

1 tablespoon chopped parsley

1 tablespoon snipped fresh chives

1 small red onion, thinly sliced

2 garlic cloves, chopped

2 tablespoons extra virgin olive oil

1 tablespoon red wine vinegar

Juice of ½ lemon

Salt and freshly ground black pepper to taste

1 can (about 400g) cannellini beans, drained and rinsed

12 radishes, thinly sliced

1 can (about 200g) tuna in water, drained

7 cherry tomatoes

1 red pepper, deseeded and thinly sliced

1 yellow pepper, deseeded and thinly sliced

1 green pepper, deseeded and thinly sliced

8 black olives

Fresh basil leaves to garnish

1. Steam the green beans until tender. Refresh under cold running water and set aside.

2. Toss the salad greens with the parsley, chives and onion in a large bowl.

3. Stir together the garlic, oil, vinegar and lemon juice in a small bowl. Season to taste with salt and pepper. Pour two-thirds of this dressing over the salad greens and toss to coat.

4. Arrange the green beans, cannellini beans, radishes, tuna, tomatoes, peppers and olives on top of the greens. Add the remaining dressing and garnish with basil.

NUTRITIONAL INFORMATION

PER SERVING: 223kcal, 19g protein, 20g carbohydrate, 8g fat, 1g saturated fat, 25mg cholesterol, 8g fibre, 310mg sodium

Rigatoni with tenderstem broccoli, cherry tomatoes and sweet garlic

SERVES 4

350g (12oz) rigatoni

8 garlic cloves

225g (8oz) tenderstem or sprouting broccoli, cut crossways into 2.5cm (1in) pieces

1 tablespoon olive oil

1 red onion, halved and thinly sliced crossways

1 yellow pepper, deseeded and cut lengthways into thin strips

2 spring onions, thinly sliced on the diagonal

75g (2¾oz) sultanas

¼ teaspoon crushed dried chillies

¼ teaspoon salt

12 cherry tomatoes, halved

Pinch of grated nutmeg

¼ teaspoon freshly ground black pepper

25g (1oz) Parmesan cheese, freshly grated

1. Cook the rigatoni with the peeled garlic cloves in boiling water according to packet instructions until al dente. Add the broccoli to the pan of pasta for the last 5 minutes of cooking. When ready, drain in a colander.

2. Meanwhile, heat the oil in a large non-stick frying pan over a moderately high heat. Add the onion, yellow pepper, spring onions, sultanas, chillies and salt. Sauté for about 5 minutes or until the vegetables are just tender. Remove the pan from the heat.

3. Return the pasta, garlic and broccoli to their empty pan. Stir in the pepper mixture, tomatoes and nutmeg. Sprinkle with the black pepper and cheese, then serve.

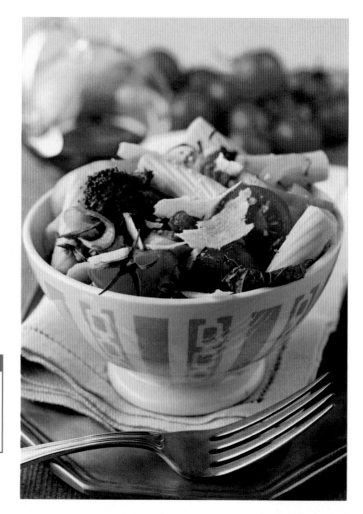

NUTRITIONAL INFORMATION

PER SERVING: 452kcal, 17g protein, 86g carbohydrate, 7g fat, 2g saturated fat, 6mg cholesterol, 6g fibre, 196mg sodium

Penne with tomato sauce and grilled aubergine

SERVES 4

1–2 aubergines, about 450g (1lb) in total, cut lengthways into 2cm (¾in) slices

½ teaspoon salt

2 tablespoons olive oil

4 garlic cloves, thinly sliced

675g (1½lb) ripe plum tomatoes, deseeded and coarsely chopped

1 teaspoon chopped fresh oregano or ½ teaspoon dried, crumbled

2 teaspoons balsamic vinegar

½ teaspoon sugar

225g (8oz) penne

25g (1oz) Parmesan cheese, freshly shaved or grated

1. Sprinkle the aubergine with ¼ teaspoon of the salt. Allow to stand for at least 30 minutes to draw out liquid.

2. Meanwhile, heat the oil in a large non-stick frying pan over a moderately low heat. Add the garlic and fry, stirring, for 1 minute. Add the tomatoes, oregano and the remaining ¼ teaspoon salt. Increase the heat to moderate and cook for about 6 minutes or just until the tomatoes are softened. Stir in the vinegar and sugar, and cook for a further 30 seconds.

3. Preheat the grill. Rinse the aubergine and pat dry. Lightly spray both sides of the slices with cooking spray. Grill for about 5 minutes on each side or until softened. Set aside to cool slightly.

4. Meanwhile, cook the pasta in boiling water according to packet instructions until al dente. Drain and toss with the tomato sauce. Coarsely chop the aubergine and add to the pasta, then stir in the cheese. Serve hot or at room temperature.

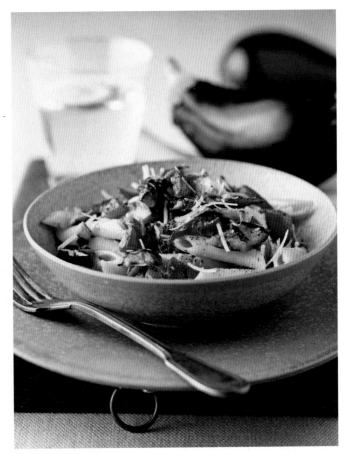

NUTRITIONAL INFORMATION
PER SERVING: 322kcal, 12g protein, 52g carbohydrate, 9g fat, 2g saturated fat, 6mg cholesterol, 6g fibre, 317mg sodium

Soba noodles with tofu and green vegetables

SERVES 4

1 tablespoon vegetable oil

4 spring onions, chopped

4 garlic cloves, crushed

1 courgette, halved
lengthways and cut across
into 5mm (¼in) slices

125ml (4fl oz) vegetable
or chicken stock, made
without salt

2 tablespoons reduced-
sodium soy sauce

2 teaspoons cornflour

1 teaspoon toasted
sesame oil

175g (6oz) extra-firm tofu,
drained and cut into cubes

175g (6oz) soba (Japanese
buckwheat noodles) or
wholemeal noodles

125g (4oz) watercress or
baby spinach leaves

2 tablespoons chopped
fresh coriander

1. Heat the vegetable oil in a large non-stick frying pan over a moderately high heat. Reserve some of the dark green parts of the spring onions to garnish. Add the garlic, courgette and the remaining spring onions to the pan. Sauté for about 5 minutes or until softened.

2. Meanwhile, whisk together the stock, soy sauce, cornflour and sesame oil in a small bowl until smooth.

3. Add the tofu and stock mixture to the pan. Bring to the boil and cook, stirring constantly, for 1–2 minutes or until the sauce thickens. Remove from the heat.

4. Cook the noodles in boiling water according to packet instructions. Drain, reserving 225ml (8fl oz) of the cooking liquid. Rinse under cold running water.

5. Combine the noodles, courgette mixture, watercress, coriander and reserved liquid in a large bowl. Toss gently, then garnish with the reserved spring onions.

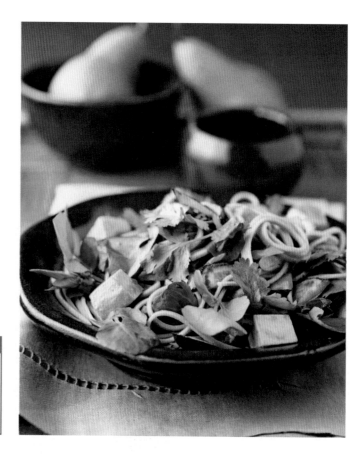

NUTRITIONAL INFORMATION

PER SERVING: 245kcal,
14g protein, 37g carbohydrate,
7g fat, 1g saturated fat,
0mg cholesterol, 2g fibre,
594mg sodium

Pineapple coleslaw

SERVES 8

450g (1lb) mixed shredded green and red cabbage and carrots

1 green pepper, deseeded and finely chopped

1 can (about 400g) pineapple pieces in natural juice

2 tablespoons reduced-fat mayonnaise

1 tablespoon wine vinegar

1 teaspoon Dijon mustard

2½ teaspoons Splenda sweetener

Salt and freshly ground black pepper

1. Put the cabbage mixture and green pepper in a large bowl. Chop the pineapple (with juice) and add to the bowl.

2. Combine the mayonnaise, vinegar, mustard, sweetener, and salt and pepper to taste in a small bowl. Add to the cabbage mixture and stir well to combine. Chill for several hours or overnight. Mix well before serving.

NUTRITIONAL INFORMATION

PER SERVING: 50kcal, 1g protein, 10g carbohydrate, 1g fat, 0.2g saturated fat, 1mg cholesterol, 1.5g fibre, 93mg sodium

Roasted carrots with rosemary

SERVES 6

450g (1lb) large carrots, peeled and cut into 5cm x 5mm (2 x ¼in) sticks

¼ teaspoon salt

1½ teaspoons olive oil

1 teaspoon finely chopped fresh rosemary or ½ teaspoon dried, crumbled

1. Preheat the oven to 200°C (400°F, gas mark 6).

2. Mound the carrots on a baking tray. Sprinkle with the salt and drizzle with the oil, then toss gently to coat. Spread out to a single layer.

3. Roast for 10 minutes. Stir in the rosemary, then continue roasting for 7–10 minutes or until just tender and lightly browned in spots.

NUTRITIONAL INFORMATION

PER SERVING: 34kcal, 0.5g protein, 6g carbohydrate, 1g fat, 0.2g saturated fat, 0mg cholesterol, 2g fibre, 101mg sodium

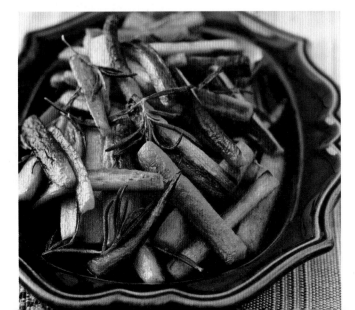

Courgette and tomato gratin

SERVES 8

100g (3½oz) seasoned dried breadcrumbs

25g (1oz) Parmesan cheese, freshly grated

1–2 teaspoons finely chopped garlic

Salt and freshly ground black pepper to taste

3–4 courgettes, peeled and cut into 5mm (¼in) slices

1 large onion, thinly sliced

4–5 large tomatoes, peeled and cut into 5mm (¼in) slices

2 tablespoons olive oil

1. Preheat the oven to 180°C (350°F, gas mark 4). Spray a large baking dish with cooking spray.

2. Stir together the breadcrumbs, cheese, garlic, and salt and pepper to taste in a medium bowl.

3. Place a layer of courgettes in the bottom of the baking dish. Add a layer of onion, then tomatoes. Sprinkle with a few tablespoons of the breadcrumb mixture. Repeat the layers, ending with tomatoes and the breadcrumb mixture. Sprinkle with the olive oil. Cover and bake for about 45 minutes or until the top is crisp and golden brown.

NUTRITIONAL INFORMATION

PER SERVING: 105kcal, 4g protein, 13g carbohydrate, 4g fat, 1g saturated fat, 3mg cholesterol, 1.5g fibre, 315mg sodium

Easy green bean casserole

SERVES 6

750g (1lb 10oz) frozen green beans

1 can (about 300g) fat-free mushroom soup

5 tablespoons skimmed milk

4 tablespoons chopped spring onions

8 table water biscuits, coarsely crushed

1. Preheat the oven to 180°C (350°F, gas mark 4).

2. Stir together the green beans, soup, milk and spring onion in a baking dish. Bake for about 30 minutes. Stir, then top with the crushed biscuits and spray with cooking spray. Bake for a further 5 minutes.

NUTRITIONAL INFORMATION

PER SERVING: 90kcal, 4g protein, 13g carbohydrate, 3g fat, 1g saturated fat, 2mg cholesterol, 5g fibre, 290mg sodium

Rosemary peas and onions

SERVES 4

175g (6oz) button or baby onions, peeled

300g (10½oz) shelled fresh or frozen peas

1 tablespoon reduced-fat spread

1 tablespoon chopped fresh rosemary

¼ teaspoon freshly ground black pepper

1. Bring 300ml (½ pint) of water to the boil in a large saucepan over a high heat. Reduce the heat to moderate, add the onions and cover. Cook for 8 minutes.

2. Add the peas, bring back to the boil and cook, covered, for 7–9 minutes.

3. Meanwhile, melt the spread in a small saucepan over a low heat. Add the rosemary and cook for 2–3 minutes.

4. Drain the peas and onions. Add the rosemary mixture and pepper, and toss gently.

NUTRITIONAL INFORMATION

PER SERVING: 90kcal, 6g protein, 12g carbohydrate, 4g fat, 0.5g saturated fat, 0mg cholesterol, 4g fibre, 25mg sodium

Steamed sesame spinach

SERVES 4

450g (1lb) fresh spinach, stalks removed

⅛ teaspoon crushed dried chillies

½ teaspoon toasted sesame oil

1 teaspoon fresh lemon juice

1 tablespoon sesame seeds, toasted

1. Place a steamer basket or rack over a pan of water and bring to the boil. Add the spinach and chillies, and steam for 3–5 minutes or until tender.

2. Transfer to a serving bowl. Add the oil and lemon juice, and toss. Sprinkle with the sesame seeds.

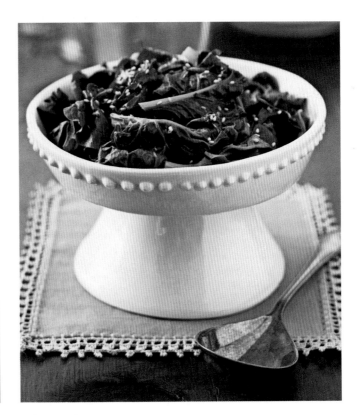

NUTRITIONAL INFORMATION

PER SERVING: 54kcal, 4g protein, 2g carbohydrate, 3g fat, 0.5g saturated fat, 0mg cholesterol, 3g fibre, 158mg sodium

Chargrilled vegetable salad

SERVES 6

1 aubergine, about 350g (12oz)

1 small fennel bulb, about 175g (6oz), trimmed

1 yellow courgette

1 green courgette

½ teaspoon salt

1 small red pepper, halved lengthways and deseeded

3 plum tomatoes, halved lengthways and deseeded

2 tablespoons olive oil

2 garlic cloves, crushed

1 teaspoon finely chopped fresh marjoram or ½ teaspoon dried, crumbled

1½ tablespoons balsamic vinegar

1. Heat a ridged cast-iron grill pan. Cut the aubergine, fennel and courgettes lengthways into 1cm (½in) slices. Sprinkle with ¼ teaspoon of the salt and spray generously with cooking spray.

2. Chargrill the pepper, skin side down, for 3–4 minutes or until blackened and blistered. Remove from the pan.

3. Chargrill the aubergine, fennel and courgettes on one side for about 4 minutes or until grill marks are dark brown but the vegetables are still very firm. Turn and chargrill the other side until browned and just tender – about 3 minutes for the courgettes and 5–6 minutes longer for the aubergine and fennel. Remove the vegetables from the pan as they are cooked.

4. Coat the cut sides of the tomatoes with cooking spray. Chargrill, cut sides down, for about 3 minutes or just until light grill marks appear. Remove from the pan.

5. Heat the oil in a small frying pan over a moderate heat. Add the garlic, marjoram and the remaining ¼ teaspoon salt. Sauté for 1 minute.

6. Peel the chargrilled pepper and cut into strips. Cut the rest of the vegetables into bite-size chunks. Transfer to a medium bowl and add the olive oil mixture and vinegar. Toss to coat. Serve at room temperature.

NUTRITIONAL INFORMATION

PER SERVING: 85kcal,
2g protein, 10g carbohydrate,
5g fat, 1g saturated fat,
0mg cholesterol, 3g fibre,
211mg sodium

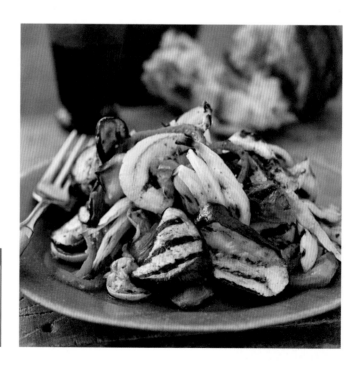

Waldorf salad

SERVES 4

115g (4oz) chopped Granny Smith or other tart dessert apples

1 tablespoon lemon juice

2 tablespoons reduced-fat mayonnaise

2 tablespoons fat-free plain yogurt

1 celery stick, chopped

40g (1½oz) raisins

2 tablespoons chopped walnuts

1. Sprinkle the apples with the lemon juice. Mix together the mayonnaise and yogurt in a small bowl.

2. Stir together the apples, celery, raisins and walnuts in a medium bowl. Add the dressing and toss to coat.

NUTRITIONAL INFORMATION

PER SERVING: 116kcal, 2g protein, 11g carbohydrate, 7g fat, 1g saturated fat, 1.5mg cholesterol, 1g fibre, 86mg sodium

Black bean and sweetcorn salad

SERVES 10

2 cans (about 400g each) black beans, drained and rinsed

1 can (about 400g) sweetcorn, drained

2 teaspoons finely chopped garlic

1 green or red pepper, deseeded and chopped

85g (3oz) finely chopped onion

125ml (4fl oz) lime juice

2 teaspoons ground cumin

2 teaspoons dried oregano

2 tablespoons chopped parsley

1 teaspoon crushed dried chillies (optional)

1. Combine the black beans, sweetcorn, garlic, pepper, onion, lime juice, cumin, oregano, parsley and chillies, if using, in a large bowl.

2. Mix well and serve chilled. (Alternatively, heat for serving.)

NUTRITIONAL INFORMATION

PER SERVING: 120kcal, 7g protein, 23g carbohydrate, 0.5g fat, 0g saturated fat, 0mg cholesterol, 4.5g fibre, 316mg sodium

German-style potato salad

SERVES 6

675g (1½lb) small new potatoes, scrubbed and quartered

½ teaspoon salt

4 turkey rashers

1 small onion, chopped

4 tablespoons cider vinegar

2 tablespoons caster sugar

1 tablespoon coarse-grain Dijon mustard

1 teaspoon olive oil

½ teaspoon freshly ground black pepper

4 tablespoons finely chopped sweet-sour gherkins

4 tablespoons finely chopped red pepper

4 tablespoon finely chopped parsley

1. Place the potatoes and enough water to cover in a large saucepan. Add ¼ teaspoon of the salt and bring to the boil. Reduce the heat and cook for 10–15 minutes or until tender. When ready, drain and keep warm.

2. Meanwhile, cut the turkey rashers across in half and cook in a large, deep non-stick frying pan until crisp. Drain on kitchen paper, then crumble. Sauté the onion in the pan juices for about 7 minutes or until golden.

3. Shake the vinegar, sugar, mustard, oil, black pepper and the remaining ¼ teaspoon salt in a jar, then whisk into the pan juices. Bring to a simmer and cook for 2 minutes. Add the potatoes, gherkins, red pepper and half of the turkey. Cook, stirring, for 2 minutes or until the potatoes are evenly coated and heated through. Sprinkle with the parsley and the remaining turkey. Serve warm or at room temperature.

NUTRITIONAL INFORMATION

PER SERVING: 132kcal, 6g protein, 25g carbohydrate, 2g fat, 0.5g saturated fat, 15mg cholesterol, 1.5g fibre, 192mg sodium

---

Scalloped potatoes

SERVES 8

4 onions, thinly sliced

175ml (4–6fl oz) chicken stock made without salt

1 can (about 400g) light evaporated milk

675g (1½lb) potatoes, peeled and sliced

Salt and freshly ground black pepper to taste

Pinch of paprika

1. Preheat the oven to 220°C (425°F, gas mark 7). Lightly spray a shallow baking dish with cooking spray.

2. Bring the onions and 125ml (4fl oz) of the stock to the boil in a non-stick frying pan over a moderate heat. Reduce the heat and simmer, stirring occasionally, for 10 minutes or until tender, adding more stock if the mixture becomes dry. Add the milk and heat for about 10 minutes.

3. Arrange half of the potatoes in the baking dish and season with salt and pepper to taste. Spoon half of the onion mixture on top. Add another layer of potatoes, then the remaining onions. Lightly season with salt and pepper and sprinkle with the paprika. Bake for 30 minutes or until lightly browned and the potatoes are tender when a fork is inserted in the middle.

NUTRITIONAL INFORMATION

PER SERVING: 135kcal, 6g protein, 23g carbohydrate, 2g fat, 1g saturated fat, 8mg cholesterol, 2g fibre, 114mg sodium

---

Irish mash with cabbage and leeks

SERVES 8

900g (2lb) small floury
  potatoes, quartered

450ml (16fl oz) chicken stock
  made without salt

450g (1lb) leeks, trimmed
  and thinly sliced

225ml (8fl oz) semi-skimmed
  milk

3 garlic cloves, crushed

1 bay leaf

1 green cabbage, about
  450g (1lb), cored and
  thinly sliced

4 tablespoons cold water

¼ teaspoon grated nutmeg

¼ teaspoon salt

¼ teaspoon white pepper

25g (1oz) unsalted butter

4 tablespoons snipped chives

1. Place the potatoes, stock and enough water to cover in a large saucepan. Bring to the boil and cook for about 20 minutes or until tender.

2. Meanwhile, combine the leeks, milk, garlic and bay leaf in another large saucepan. Cover and bring to the boil. Reduce the heat and simmer for 15–20 minutes or until the leeks are softened. Drain, reserving the leeks, milk and garlic separately. Discard the bay leaf.

3. In the same saucepan, combine the cabbage and water. Cover and bring to a gentle boil. Cook for 10–15 minutes or until tender, then drain. Squeeze dry and chop finely.

4. Drain the potatoes and transfer to a large bowl. Add the milk and garlic, and mash. Stir in the leeks, cabbage, nutmeg, salt, pepper and butter. Top with the chives.

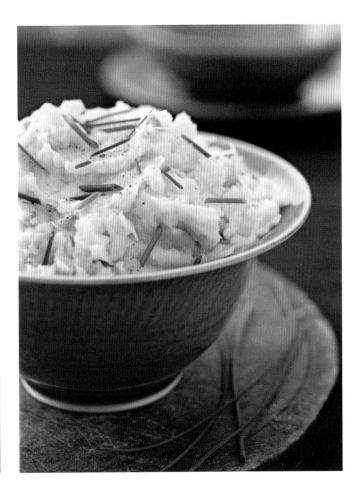

NUTRITIONAL INFORMATION

PER SERVING: 148kcal,
5g protein, 25g carbohydrate,
4g fat, 2g saturated fat,
8mg cholesterol, 4g fibre,
104mg sodium

Praline-sweet potato casserole

SERVES 12

675g (1½lb) sweet potatoes

4 egg whites

½ teaspoon salt

1 teaspoon mixed spice

100g (3½oz) soft brown sugar

25g (1oz) pecan nuts, chopped

4 tablespoons plain flour

2 tablespoons reduced-fat spread

1. Preheat the oven to 180°C (350°F, gas mark 4). Bake the sweet potatoes for about 45 minutes or until tender. When cool enough to handle, peel off the skin.

2. Lightly grease (or spray with cooking spray) a large, shallow baking dish or gratin dish.

3. Combine the sweet potatoes, egg whites, salt and mixed spice in a food processor or blender and process until smooth. Spoon into the baking dish.

4. Stir together the brown sugar, pecans, flour and spread in a medium bowl. Lightly sprinkle over the sweet potato mixture. Spray the top with butter-flavoured cooking spray. Bake for about 30 minutes or until lightly browned.

NUTRITIONAL INFORMATION

PER SERVING: 129kcal, 2g protein, 25g carbohydrate, 3g fat, 0.5g saturated fat, 0mg cholesterol, 1.5g fibre, 142mg sodium

Sage and onion stuffing

SERVES 6

90g (3¼oz) finely chopped celery

125g (4½oz) chopped onions

1½ tablespoons chopped parsley

2 teaspoons dried sage

150g (5½oz) stale bread, cut into small cubes

500ml (18fl oz) chicken stock made without salt

1. Preheat the oven to 180°C (350°F, gas mark 4). Spray a baking dish with cooking spray.

2. Spray a medium non-stick frying pan with cooking spray. Add the celery and onions and cook, stirring occasionally, until tender. Stir in the parsley and sage.

3. Place the bread cubes in the baking dish and top with the onion mixture. Drizzle with 400ml (14fl oz) of the stock. Toss gently to combine. Add the remaining stock if the mixture is too dry. Bake for about 30 minutes or until lightly browned.

NUTRITIONAL INFORMATION

PER SERVING: 70kcal, 3g protein, 13g carbohydrate, 1g fat, 0g saturated fat, 0mg cholesterol, 1g fibre, 305mg sodium

Lemon barley with sultanas

SERVES 8

2 tablespoons olive oil

2 onions, finely chopped

3 celery sticks, finely chopped

200g (7oz) pearl barley, rinsed

600ml (1 pint) chicken stock made without salt

1 teaspoon finely grated lemon zest

½ teaspoon dried oregano

Pinch of salt

Pinch of freshly ground black pepper

2 tablespoons sunflower seeds

1 tablespoon fresh lemon juice

40g (1½oz) sultanas

2 tablespoons chopped parsley

1. Heat the oil in a large, heavy saucepan over a moderate heat. Add the onions and celery, and sauté, stirring, for about 7 minutes or until softened and lightly browned. Stir in the barley until coated with oil. Add the stock, lemon zest, oregano, salt and pepper.

2. Bring to the boil, then reduce the heat. Cover and simmer, stirring occasionally, for about 40 minutes or until the barley is nearly cooked and almost all of the liquid has been absorbed.

3. Meanwhile, toast the sunflower seeds in a non-stick frying pan over moderate heat, stirring frequently or shaking the pan, until golden brown. Transfer to a plate.

4. Stir the lemon juice and sultanas into the barley mixture. Cover, remove from the heat and allow to stand for about 5 minutes. Gently stir in the sunflower seeds and parsley until combined, then serve.

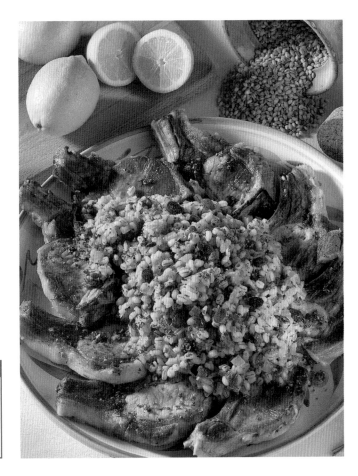

NUTRITIONAL INFORMATION
PER SERVING: 170kcal, 6g protein, 28g carbohydrate, 5g fat, 1g saturated fat, 0mg cholesterol, 1g fibre, 149mg sodium

Bulghur wheat with spring vegetables

SERVES 6

200g (7oz) bulghur wheat

3 tablespoons fresh lemon
juice

1 teaspoon salt

½ teaspoon freshly ground
black pepper

2 tablespoons olive oil

2 leeks, halved lengthways
and cut across into 2.5cm
(1in) pieces

2 garlic cloves, crushed

12 asparagus spears, cut into
5cm (2in) pieces

150g (5½oz) frozen peas

4 tablespoons chopped fresh
mint

1. Put the bulghur wheat in a large heatproof bowl and pour
over enough boiling water to cover. Leave to soak for
about 30 minutes or until the bulghur is tender. Drain
well in a large, fine-meshed sieve.

2. Combine the lemon juice, salt, pepper and 1 tablespoon
of the oil in a large bowl and whisk to mix. Add the
bulghur wheat and fluff with a fork.

3. Heat the remaining 1 tablespoon of oil in a large frying
pan over a moderate heat. Add the leeks and garlic, and
cook for about 5 minutes or until the leeks are tender.
Transfer to the bowl.

4. Place a steamer basket or rack over a pan of water and
bring to the boil. Add the asparagus and steam for about
4 minutes or until tender. Add the peas during the final
30 seconds of steaming. Add the asparagus, peas and
mint to the bulghur wheat and toss to combine. Serve at
room temperature or chilled.

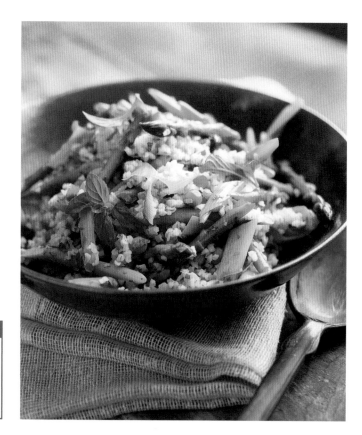

NUTRITIONAL INFORMATION

PER SERVING: 185kcal,
6g protein, 32g carbohydrate,
5g fat, 1g saturated fat,
0mg cholesterol, 2.5g fibre,
330mg sodium

Hearty turkey chilli

SERVES 4

225g (8oz) lean minced turkey

1 onion, chopped

1 small green pepper, deseeded and chopped

1 tablespoon mild chilli powder, or to taste

1 teaspoon dry mustard

1 can (about 400g) tomatoes

125ml (4fl oz) tomato sauce

1 garlic clove, crushed

55g (2oz) mushrooms, sliced

2 cans (about 400g each) red kidney beans, drained and rinsed

1. Spray a large frying pan with cooking spray. Add the turkey and cook until browned. Drain off any fat.

2. Add the onion, pepper, chilli powder and mustard, and cook for 5 minutes.

3. Add the tomatoes with their juice, tomato sauce, garlic, mushrooms and beans. Simmer for 30–45 minutes.

NUTRITIONAL INFORMATION
PER SERVING: 260kcal, 24g protein, 34g carbohydrate, 4g fat, 1g saturated fat, 48mg cholesterol, 10g fibre, 806mg sodium

Spiced pumpkin and bacon soup

SERVES 4

1 tablespoon olive oil

200g (7oz) onions, sliced

1.3kg (3lb) pumpkin, peeled, deseeded and cut into chunks

125g (4½oz) well trimmed smoked back bacon, diced

1 tablespoon ground cumin

750ml (1 pint 7fl oz) vegetable stock, made without salt

Salt and freshly ground black pepper

Sprigs of fresh coriander to garnish

1. Heat the oil in a saucepan and add the onions. Stir to coat them with oil, then cover and cook over a low heat, stirring occasionally, for 5–10 minutes or until they start to soften.

2. Add the pumpkin, bacon and cumin to the pan. Stir, then cover and simmer for 10 minutes, stirring occasionally.

3. Add the stock, raise the heat and bring to the boil. Lower the heat and simmer, uncovered, for 20 minutes or until the pumpkin is tender.

4. Purée the soup with a hand-held blender or in a food processor. Season to taste. Serve hot, garnished with coriander and black pepper and accompanied by crusty bread rolls, if you like.

VARIATION: if you cannot get fresh pumpkin, use 1 can (about 425g) unsweetened pumpkin, which is usually found on the canned fruit shelves in supermarkets.

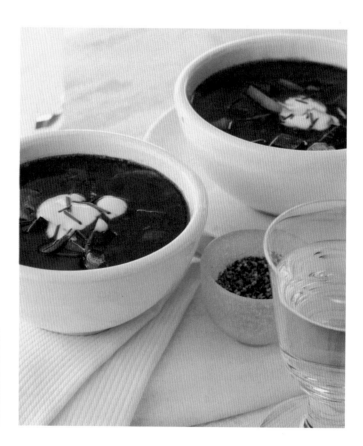

NUTRITIONAL INFORMATION

PER SERVING: 137kcal, 10g protein, 12g carbohydrate, 6g fat, 1.5g saturated fat, 5mg cholesterol, 4.5g fibre, 692mg sodium

Lemony lentil soup

SERVES 4

1 tablespoon olive oil

3 garlic cloves, coarsely
chopped

250g (9oz) onions, coarsely
chopped

250g (9oz) red lentils, rinsed
and drained

1.2 litres (2 pints) chicken
or vegetable stock, made
without salt

1 teaspoon ground
coriander

½ teaspoon ground cumin

Juice of 1 lemon

4 wafer-thin slices of lemon

Salt and freshly ground
black pepper

1. Heat the olive oil in a heavy-based saucepan. Add the
garlic and onions and cook over a moderate heat for
6–7 minutes or until they turn a rich brown colour,
stirring frequently to prevent them from sticking.

2. Add the lentils and cook for a further 1–2 minutes. Add
the stock, raise the heat and bring the soup to the boil.
Reduce the heat, cover and simmer for 15–20 minutes
or until the lentils are almost soft.

3. Place a small non-stick frying pan over a high heat and
add the coriander and cumin. Dry-fry for 1–2 minutes
or until their aroma rises. Add them to the soup.

4. Raise the heat under the soup, add the lemon juice and
lemon slices, and season to taste. Leave the soup to
simmer for a further 5 minutes. Sprinkle with a little
black pepper before serving.

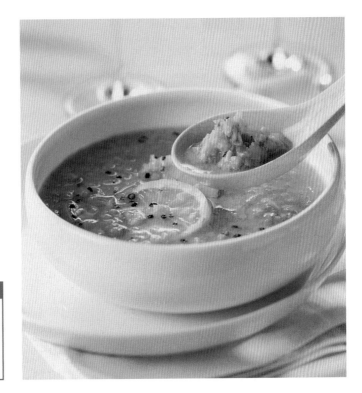

NUTRITIONAL INFORMATION

PER SERVING: 300kcal, 25g
protein, 42g carbohydrate,
6g fat, 1g saturated fat,
0mg cholesterol, 4.5g fibre,
24mg sodium

Winter slimming soup

2 cans (about 400g each) chopped tomatoes

450ml (16fl oz) tomato passata

1 litre (1¾ pints) water

4 beef stock cubes

1–2 garlic cloves, chopped

1 large turnip

1 green pepper

½ celery stick

1 large onion

1 courgette

2 large carrots

1 small cabbage, shredded

225g (8oz) fresh or frozen green beans

115g (4oz) thawed frozen chopped spinach

1 teaspoon dried thyme

1 teaspoon dried oregano

1 bay leaf

Salt and freshly ground black pepper

1. Combine the tomatoes with their juice, tomato passata, water, stock cubes and garlic in a large saucepan. Chop the turnip, pepper, celery, onion, courgette and carrots into large pieces and add to the pan. Bring to the boil.

2. Simmer gently for about 1 hour or until the vegetables are soft but still firm.

3. Stir in the cabbage, beans, spinach, thyme, oregano, bay leaf, and salt and pepper to taste. Simmer until all the vegetables are tender. Discard the bay leaf before serving. (The soup is suitable for freezing; reheat from frozen.)

NUTRITIONAL INFORMATION

PER SERVING: 50kcal, 3g protein, 11g carbohydrate, 1g fat, 0.1g saturated fat, 0mg cholesterol, 3g fibre, 400mg sodium

---

Breads

Hearty bread-machine loaf

MAKES 12 SLICES

300ml (½ pint) water

1½ teaspoons salt

1 tablespoon Splenda
sweetener

2 tablespoons skimmed milk
powder

2 tablespoons vegetable oil

40g (1½oz) rolled oats

2 tablespoons wheat germ

3 tablespoons chopped
walnuts

55g (2oz) wholemeal flour

350g (12oz) white bread flour

2 teaspoons easy-blend dried
yeast

1. Combine the ingredients in a bread machine following
the manufacturer's instructions.

2. Use the white or wholemeal bread setting for a 700g
(1½lb) loaf.

NUTRITIONAL INFORMATION

PER SLICE: 206kcal, 6g protein, 32g carbohydrate, 5g fat,
0.5g saturated fat, 0mg cholesterol, 2g fibre, 61mg sodium

Banana bran muffins

MAKES 12 MUFFINS

35g (1¼oz) branflake cereal

350g (12oz) mashed banana
or unsweetened puréed
apple

4 tablespoons skimmed milk

115g (4oz) wholemeal flour

40g (1½oz) rolled oats

1 tablespoon baking powder

½ teaspoon bicarbonate of
soda

1 tablespoon clear honey

1 tablespoon molasses or dark
treacle

1 teaspoon ground cinnamon

2 egg whites or 1 whole egg

1. Preheat the oven to 200°C (400°F, gas mark 6). Spray a
12-cup muffin tin with cooking spray or insert paper
liners in the cups.

2. Combine the cereal, banana and milk in a large bowl.
Allow to stand for about 5 minutes.

3. Add the flour, oats, baking powder, bicarbonate of soda,
honey, molasses or dark treacle, cinnamon and egg whites
or whole egg and stir until just combined.

4. Spoon the mixture into the tins and bake for 20 minutes.

NUTRITIONAL INFORMATION

PER MUFFIN: 100kcal, 3g protein, 21g carbohydrate, 0.7g fat,
0.1g saturated fat, 0mg cholesterol, 2g fibre, 243mg sodium

Desserts

Lemon-lime yogurt mousse

SERVES 8

1 sachet sugar-free lemon and lime jelly

500g (1lb 2oz) fat-free or very-low-fat lemon or lime yogurt

225ml (8fl oz) whipping cream, whipped until thick

1. Pour 150ml (5fl oz) boiling water into a medium bowl, add the jelly and stir to dissolve. Allow to cool.

2. Stir in the yogurt until blended, then fold in three-quarters of the cream.

3. Chill for about 30 minutes. Serve topped with the remaining cream.

NUTRITIONAL INFORMATION

PER SERVING: 138kcal, 5g protein, 4g carbohydrate, 11g fat, 7g saturated fat, 30mg cholesterol, 0g fibre, 30mg sodium

Chocolate–banana pudding parfait

SERVES 4

1 packet no-sugar-added chocolate instant pudding mix

300ml (½ pint) semi-skimmed milk

2 bananas, sliced

Light aerosol cream

1 teaspoon shaved chocolate

1. Make up the pudding with the milk according to packet instructions. Layer with the banana in 4 dessert glasses.

2. Add a dollop of cream to each parfait and garnish with the chocolate. Serve immediately.

NUTRITIONAL INFORMATION

PER SERVING: 146kcal, 4g protein, 22g carbohydrate, 4.5g fat, 3.5g saturated fat, 0.7mg cholesterol, 3g fibre, 200mg sodium

Hot plum sauce

SERVES 4

450g (1lb) ripe dessert plums, halved and stoned

150ml (5fl oz) orange juice

Large pinch of ground cinnamon

Large pinch of ground cloves

1 teaspoon light soft brown sugar, or to taste

1. Combine the plums, orange juice and spices in a saucepan. Bring slowly to the boil, then simmer gently for 10 minutes or until very soft.

2. Press the fruit mixture through a sieve into a bowl. Stir in the sugar. If necessary, return the sauce to the pan and reheat gently before serving.

NUTRITIONAL INFORMATION

PER SERVING: 47kcal, 0.8g protein, 11g carbohydrate, 0.1g fat, 0g saturated fat, 0.5mg cholesterol, 0.5g fibre, 5mg sodium

Lemon angel cake with strawberries

SERVES 12

550g (1¼lb) frozen strawberries, thawed

125ml (4fl oz) orange juice

12 large egg whites, at room temperature

1¼ teaspoons cream of tartar

½ teaspoon salt

250g (9oz) caster sugar

3 tablespoons grated lemon zest

1 teaspoon vanilla extract

140g (5oz) plain flour

1. Combine the strawberries and orange juice in a large bowl. Set aside in the fridge.

2. Preheat the oven to 160°C (325°F, gas mark 3). Beat the egg whites with the cream of tartar and salt in a tabletop electric mixer until foamy. Gradually beat in the sugar, 2 tablespoons at a time, until thick, soft peaks form. Beat in the lemon zest and vanilla.

3. Gently fold in the flour, in four batches, until evenly incorporated. Spoon into an ungreased 25cm (10in) non-stick angel cake or tube tin. Bake for about 50 minutes or until the top springs back when lightly pressed.

4. Invert the tin over the neck of a bottle to cool. When the cake is cold, remove by running a palette knife around the edge and centre and turning right side up on a plate. Serve with the strawberries and juice.

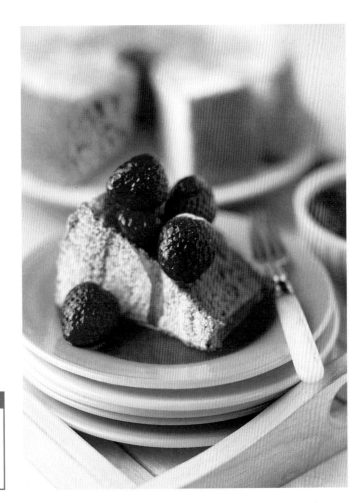

NUTRITIONAL INFORMATION

PER SERVING: 150kcal, 4.5g protein, 34g carbohydrate, 0.2g fat, 0g saturated fat, 0mg cholesterol, 1g fibre, 153mg sodium

Tropical fruit pudding

SERVES 10

1 packet no-sugar-added
vanilla instant
pudding mix

300ml (½ pint) semi-
skimmed milk

2 cans (about 400g each)
tropical fruit salad in
natural juice, drained

1 can (about 400g)
pineapple pieces in natural
juice, drained and
chopped

1 can (about 400g)
mandarin oranges in
natural juice, drained

125ml (4fl oz) whipping
cream, whipped
until thick

1. Combine the pudding mix and milk in a large bowl and whisk until smooth.

2. Fold in the fruit and cream. Chill until ready to serve, but within 2 hours of making.

NUTRITIONAL INFORMATION

PER SERVING: 150kcal, 2g protein, 19g carbohydrate, 7g fat, 5g saturated fat, 15mg cholesterol, 0.7g fibre, 105mg sodium

Peach crisp

SERVES 9

700g (1lb 9oz) sliced fresh,
ripe but firm peaches or
thawed frozen peaches

1 teaspoon ground
cinnamon

40g (1½oz) rolled oats

2 tablespoons chopped
walnuts

40g (1½oz) digestive
biscuits, crushed

100g (3½oz) soft brown
sugar

2 tablespoons reduced-fat
spread

1. Preheat the oven to 180°C (350°F, gas mark 4).

2. Place the peaches in a 20cm (8in) square baking dish and sprinkle with the cinnamon.

3. For the topping, stir together the oats, walnuts, biscuit crumbs and brown sugar in a medium bowl. Rub in the spread until crumbly. Scatter evenly over the peaches.

4. Bake for about 45 minutes or until the top is crisp and golden brown.

NUTRITIONAL INFORMATION

PER SERVING: 140kcal, 2g protein, 23g carbohydrate, 5g fat, 1g saturated fat, 2mg cholesterol, 2g fibre, 56mg sodium

Pear and redcurrant lattice

SERVES 6

3 sheets filo pastry, each
30 x 50cm (12 x 20in),
about 90g (3¼oz)
in total

20g (¾oz) unsalted butter,
melted

Filling

2 tablespoons redcurrant
jelly

1 teaspoon lemon juice

3 ripe but firm pears,
about 175g (6oz)
each, peeled and
thinly sliced

125g (4½oz) redcurrants,
thawed if frozen

40g (1½oz) ground almonds

1. Preheat the oven to 200°C (400°F, gas mark 6). Put a baking sheet into the oven to heat.

2. To make the filling, combine the redcurrant jelly and lemon juice in a medium saucepan and heat gently until melted. Remove from the heat. Add the pears and toss gently to coat. Stir in the redcurrants.

3. Lay out two sheets of filo on top of each other (keep the third sheet covered to prevent it from drying out). Cut into quarters. Separate the eight pieces and brush lightly with butter. Use to line a 23cm (9in) loose-bottomed, non-stick flan tin, overlapping them slightly and tucking in the edges.

4. Sprinkle the almonds over the bottom of the pastry case. Top with the fruit mixture, spreading it evenly. Cut the remaining sheet of filo into strips 2cm (¾in) wide, twist gently and arrange in a lattice over the filling, tucking in the ends neatly.

5. Place the tin on the hot baking sheet and bake the tart for 15–20 minutes or until the pastry is crisp and golden brown. Serve warm.

NUTRITIONAL INFORMATION
PER SERVING: 155kcal, 3g protein, 22g carbohydrate, 7g fat, 1g saturated fat, 7mg cholesterol, 2g fibre, 24mg sodium

Berry-filled sponge flans

SERVES 8

2 tablespoons sugar-free
high-fruit-content spread

150g (5½oz) blueberries,
sliced strawberries or
raspberries

175g (6oz) low-fat fruit
yogurt (same flavour
as fruit used)

175g (6oz) plain Greek
yogurt

8 individual sponge flan
cases

1. Place the fruit spread in a small dish and microwave for 1 minute to soften. Mix with the berries in a medium bowl to coat evenly.

2. Stir together the fruit yogurt and Greek yogurt in a small bowl. Divide among the sponge flan cases and top with the berry mixture.

NUTRITIONAL INFORMATION
PER SERVING: 217kcal, 7g protein, 37g carbohydrate, 6g fat, 2g saturated fat, 5mg cholesterol, 0.5g fibre, 71mg sodium

Recipe index

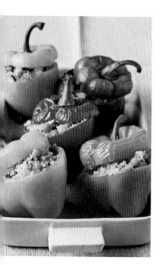

couscous-stuffed peppers 224

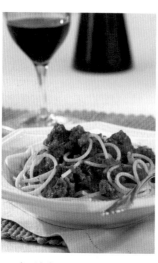

spaghetti bolognese 117

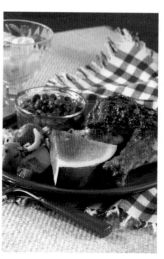

'fried' chicken 112

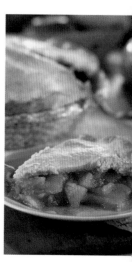

apple pie 125

peppers
  black bean and
    sweetcorn salad 233
  chargrilled vegetable
    salad 232
  couscous-stuffed
    peppers 224
  fettuccine in cream
    sauce 120
  garden beef stir-fry
    with hoisin sauce 218
  German-style potato
    salad 234
  hearty turkey chilli 239
  pineapple coleslaw 229
  prawn and vegetable
    stir-fry 222
  rigatoni with
    tenderstem broccoli,
    cherry tomatoes and
    sweet garlic 226
  steak roulade with
    spinach, carrots and
    pepper 215
  tuna salad provençale
    225
  vegetarian pizza 114
  winter slimming soup
    242
pineapple
  pineapple coleslaw 229
  tropical fruit pudding
    246
plums: hot plum sauce
    244
pork
  barbecued pork 'ribs'
    123
  pork fillet with honey-
    mustard sauce 217
potatoes
  German-style potato
    salad 234
  Irish mash with
    cabbage and leeks 235

mashed potatoes 112
  oven chips 109
  scalloped potatoes 234
prawn and vegetable
  stir-fry 222
pumpkin: spiced
  pumpkin and bacon
  soup 240

S
sage and onion stuffing
  236
salads
  black bean and
    sweetcorn salad 233
  chargrilled vegetable
    salad 232
  German-style potato
    salad 234
  tuna salad provençale
    225
  Waldorf salad 233
seafood see fish; shellfish
shellfish
  crab and artichoke rice
    223
  prawn and vegetable
    stir-fry 222
soups
  lemony lentil soup 241
  spiced pumpkin and
    bacon soup 240
  winter slimming soup
    242
spinach
  steak roulade with
    spinach, carrots and
    pepper 215
  steamed sesame
    spinach 231
  vegetarian pizza 114
  winter slimming soup
    242
sweet potatoes
  braised ham with sweet

potatoes and apples
  216
praline-sweet potato
  casserole 236
sweetcorn
  black bean and
    sweetcorn salad 233
  prawn and vegetable
    stir-fry 222
  Tex-Mex turkey
    casserole 221

T
tofu
  marbled cheesecake 126
  soba noodles with tofu
    and green vegetables
    228
tomatoes
  barbecued chicken 219
  chargrilled vegetable
    salad 232
  chicken Marsala 220
  courgette and tomato
    gratin 230
  hearty turkey chilli 239
  penne with tomato
    sauce and grilled
    aubergine 227
  rigatoni with
    tenderstem broccoli,
    cherry tomatoes and
    sweet garlic 226
  spaghetti bolognese
    117
  winter slimming soup
    242
turkey
  German-style potato
    salad 234
  hamburgers 109
  hearty turkey chilli 239
  Tex-Mex turkey
    casserole 221
  turkey enchiladas 122

General index